CREATE HEALTH WITH YOUR SEXUAL ENERGY

IRÉNE ANDERSSON

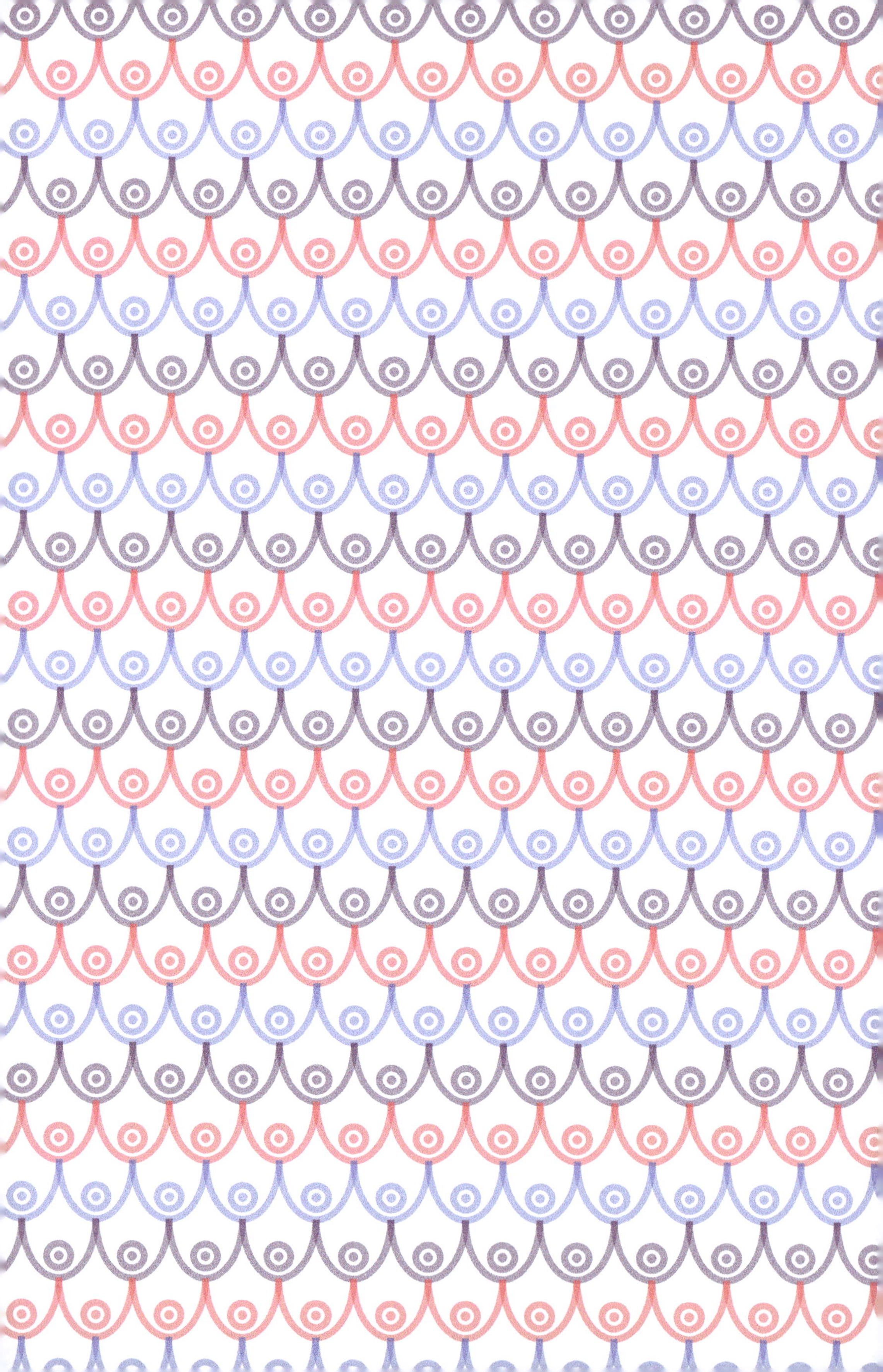

CREATE HEALTH
with your
SEXUAL ENERGY

The Tao Approach to Women's Well-Being

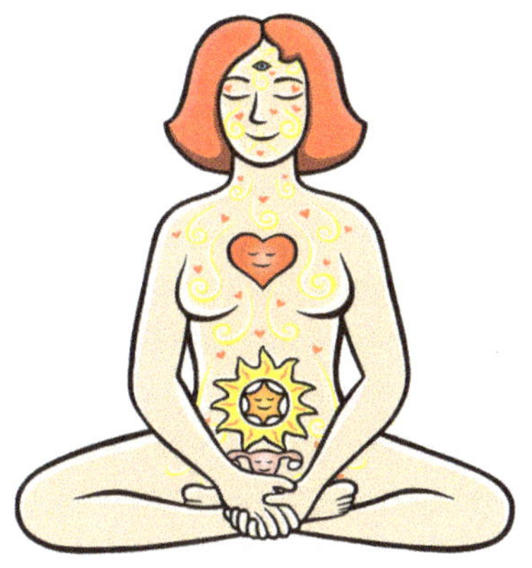

Illustrations: Lisa C. Larsson
Translation: Johan Badh

IRÉNE ANDERSSON

Also by the author:

Create Health with Your Sexual Energy: The Tao Approach to Men's Well-Being, 2020

Create Health with Your Sexual Energy: The Tao Approach to Women's Well-Being

© Iréne Andersson. Procreative AB, Stockholm, 2020.
www.bodycoach.nu
www.pelvicfloorawareness.com

Original title: Kvinnans Tao: Vägen till glädje, njutning och livsenergi!
© Iréne Andersson. Stockholm, Sweden 2011, 2016.
Publisher: ProCreative AB

The author does not provide any medical advice or prescribe the use of any exercise as a treatment for any disorder, and does not take responsibility for possible injuries while performing these exercises. As always, wrong practice, as well as inaccurate or inadequate exercise, can cause unwanted effects to some people. In case of ailments, pain or insecurity, it is recommended to seek professional help. The exercises are also not intended to cure disease, but are designed to create opportunities for recovery, self-awareness and development.

Tao is spelled Tao according to Wales-Giles, which created a method of transliterating Chinese characters into the Latin alphabet. The method was developed during the 19th century, but is often replaced by the pinyin method, and Tao is then spelled Dao. In this text, the spelling Tao is generally used, except in some Chinese book titles.

Text: Iréne Andersson
Illustrations: Lisa C. Larsson, www.tecknarlisa.com
Layout & cover: Ann-Sofie Hammarström, www.lillablatornet.se
Translation: Johan Badh

ISBN 978-91-981931-6-9   P o D
ISBN 978-91-981931-7-6   e-book

FORWORD

by Deborah Sundahl
June, 2020

Recent discoveries in Neuroscience have ushered in a new era of how to view our health, how we approach our health and how we maintain our health, including our approach to disease. We now know that our emotions affect changes in the very molecules of our body, which in turn cause changes to our health. The state of our internal environment from the food we eat, the physical movements we make each day, the emotions we feel and the thoughts we think can actually turn gene markers on and off. The control of our health is in our own hands on a daily basis.

Rather than depend on external sources to interpret our health and produce products to care for our bodies, this new approach to health relies on our internal resources. To help us pivot from outward reliance to inner reserves, Irene Andersson translated from Swedish her modern health and sexuality manual for women which uses the framework of Taoist theory. The energetic use of sexuality is the key component for Taoism's very personal approach to understanding at a deeper level one's health, and how to maintain its balance, and therefore its integrity, over one's lifetime.

To do this, Irene guides you inside your body (not outside) through practices that access the wisdom of the body, like finding ways to recognize and connect with your body's emotional inner balance system. You learn correct and important female genital anatomy that is rarely taught to us in the western world, and you discover these truths in your very own lovely vulva, such as the new science on the female prostate. Orgasm and the sexual fluids secreted by the erotic body have fascinating health benefits, including the new discovery of female ejaculation.

If that isn't enough, Irene shares her painstaking research and her unique, practical approach to making friends with our pelvic floor. Through hands-on practices, we learn in our own body what it means to bring back into our awareness this foundation of our physical, emotional, and spiritual center of the body. The pelvic floor muscles' natural state of being is a creative wellspring and a fount intuitive reasoning - a veritable bowl of self-confidence and happiness when aligned. Irene Andersson's unique approach of inner awareness to understand pelvic floor pain and repair equilibrium to its muscles and nerves offers a fresh and empowering alternative to restoring pelvic floor wellness versus employing outer intervention.

Sexual energy is the rocket fuel for building the cornerstones of inner generated health. Fortunately, the past 50 years have seen major changes in lifting sexuality out of its cultural taboo, religious shame state and banishment from every corner of life. Rescued only recently by psychology and sexology scientists, and advocated by sex therapists, counselors and educators, we know now that 90% of sexuality problems are not medical issues but only a lack of access to sexuality information and resources, support and validation, and skill-building.

While porn today has far too great an influence on our high school and college dating behavior, and adult lovemaking beds, individuals who can look under the covers of the dominate society have discovered a beautiful world of adult sex education and its supporting sexology science and psychology framework. It is this very influential world of which I refer and to which Irene Andersson has added another groundbreaking sexuality book.

Create Health with Your Sexual Energy: A Taoist Approach to Women's Well-Being shows us how to treat our body and understand our body as a biological and not mechanical mechanism, and in the doing create amazing health benefits, along with a deeper understanding of a sexuality that is utilized for health and well-being and not solely for pleasure.

Deborah Sundahl,

Author, Female Ejaculation and The G-Spot,

Seminar Speaker and Workshop Teacher

CONTENT

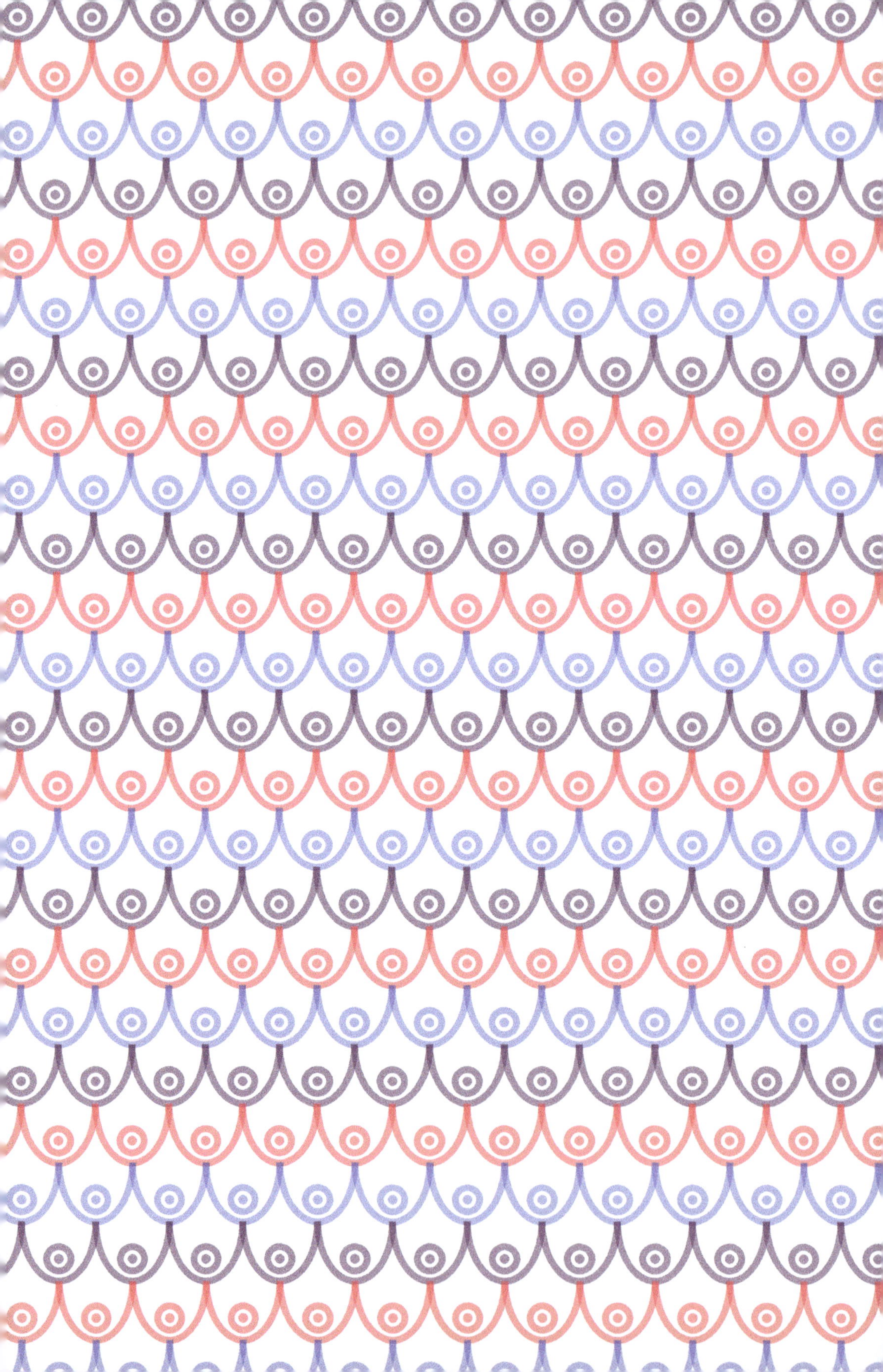

PREFACE

Besides a never-ending interest and curiosity about the human consciousness, my driving forces for writing this book have been several. Taoism is an incredibly inspiring wisdom and the power of the Taoist practices have been constantly repeated. That I also got to meet Taoist masters who had abilities far beyond the ordinary, and far from what I had previously imagined, has increased my belief in what is possible. This has also strengthened my own dedication to go deeper into the practice and exploration of myself. Moreover, I have experienced the magic of healing in my own body several times. Through the knowledge of Taoism, I also had previous mystical experiences and connections in my body explained.

Over the years I have perceived quite a bit of confusion regarding the woman's erogenous zones and erotic flows. Therefore, it became part of my mission to shed light on this, not the least because Tao points out the importance of understanding our body as a way to understand ourselves. Imagine that it was not until the mid 1990s that the size of the clitoris became widely known and that many still do not accept the fact that a woman can ejaculate. This together with dogma and disinterest has contributed to the disinformation. And this in turn is fascinating in itself, because as we know, we, as human beings, are all interested in sex. But now the time has come for the woman's sex and erogenous potential to rise into our shared consciousness and stretch our imaginations.

I have for a long time been fascinated by these fruitful Taoist tools and exercises for women. Since the mid 1990's I have used these exercises to explore and nurture myself. My own exploration has continually increased my curiosity and at the same time strengthened my desire to continue to grow as a human being, and it has also increased my desire to share my knowledge. Over the years I have guided many women and I never cease to be surprised by the power of the exercises. My respect and confidence in the self-healing abilities of the body and mind have been empowered and I perceive it to be my task to help create space for that power to grow. To be able to share these uplifting Taoist exercises with sexual Qigong for women has made it all the more inspiring and satisfying.

The exercises presented here are primarily inspired by various Taoist teachings and by my many Qigong teachers; Andrew Fretwell, David Verdesi, Mantak Chia and Wang Ting Jun. Other sources of inspiration for this book are the things I've learnt from my work as a body therapist and coach, my experience of Yoga, Tantra, shamanic body dearmoring and Quodoushka, along with my time in different centers in India. I mix Taoist theory and modern research regarding the female anatomy and erotic potential, with mine and others people's experiences and studies in alternative therapies as well as conventionally taught medicine.

With my books, "Create Health with Your Sexual Energy", for both women's and men's well-being", I hope to contribute to more acceptance, understanding and peace between the sexes. With greater balance of the masculine and feminine inside of us we can create more balance outside of us in our relationships and therefore in the world. My wish is to encourage women to love their bodies, reclaim their ability to orgasm and pleasure and to recapture the power of their wombs and realize their true dreams.

In this English version some improvements and refinements have been done from the Swedish original.

Irene Andersson, Stockholm 2020

INTRODUCTION

This book, on womens well-being, gives you access to a reliable place of recovery, joy and development; a space within yourself where you can lay the foundation for better health. You will gain a greater awareness of yourself, your body and your sexual energy. You will also get to know your feminine essence and increase your ability of sexual pleasure.

> **Create Health with Your Sexual Energy** *contains knowledge and exercises that help you find the path to your naturalness and highest potential.*

One of the teachings of Taoism is that we all have an amazing inherent potential inside of us that can be trained and which helps us grow. However, even if the seed of a plant contains the entire code of the flower, it also needs care, good conditions and nutrition to fully blossom. This book contains knowledge and practices that help you find the path to your naturalness and highest potential. By cultivating your sexual energy, you will learn how to create intimacy with yourself and develop integrity and confidence in your feelings and intuition. For women, this process means that you learn to reclaim your right to your body, your birthright to feel pleasure, orgasm and self-love. Through the exercises in this book you train yourself to cultivate your sexual capacity as well as your awareness of yourself as a human being and a woman. A pleasant side effect is also an elevated vitality, health and well-being.

From theory to exercises

This book begins with a section on Taoist theory, Qigong, sexual Qigong and what is meant by sexual energy. Then follows a description of important concepts and principles. It is equally important to learn how to perform a certain technique as it is to understand the teachings behind it. Then follows a review of the female anatomy and her erotic flows, since it is regarded as a basis for exploring the female essence, according to the Tao. Taoism also emphasizes the body as the instrument you have at your disposal in the exploration and development of yourself. The more knowledge and understanding you have about how you work the better. The final chapter of theory is about life cycles, menopause and stress. Finally comes the practices especially created for women.

The spine and directions for movement

To better understand descriptions of the location of different organs and points, we will go through the spine and directions for movement.

The spine consists of 33 vertebrae, top to bottom:

- 7 neck vertebrae counted from the top of the skull base. They are called cervical vertebrae and are termed C1-C7.
- 12 chest vertebrae, each with connected ribs. They are called thoracic vertebrae and are termed T1-T12.
- 5 vertebrae in the lower back. They are called lumbar vertebrae and are termed L1-L5.
- 5 vertebrae, grown together into the sacrum.
- 4 vertebrae, grown together into the tailbone.
- At the front of the pelvis is the pubic bone.

All movement in the exercises are described in the same way, no matter if you are standing, sitting or laying down.

- Forward intends toward the stomach.
- Backward intends toward the back.
- Down intends toward the feet.
- Up intends toward the head.

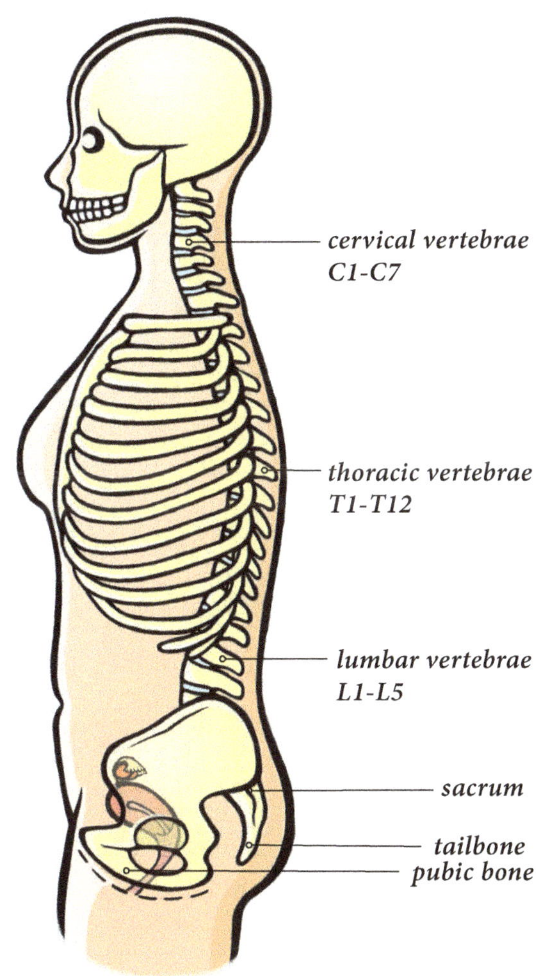
cervical vertebrae
C1-C7
thoracic vertebrae
T1-T12
lumbar vertebrae
L1-L5
sacrum
tailbone
pubic bone

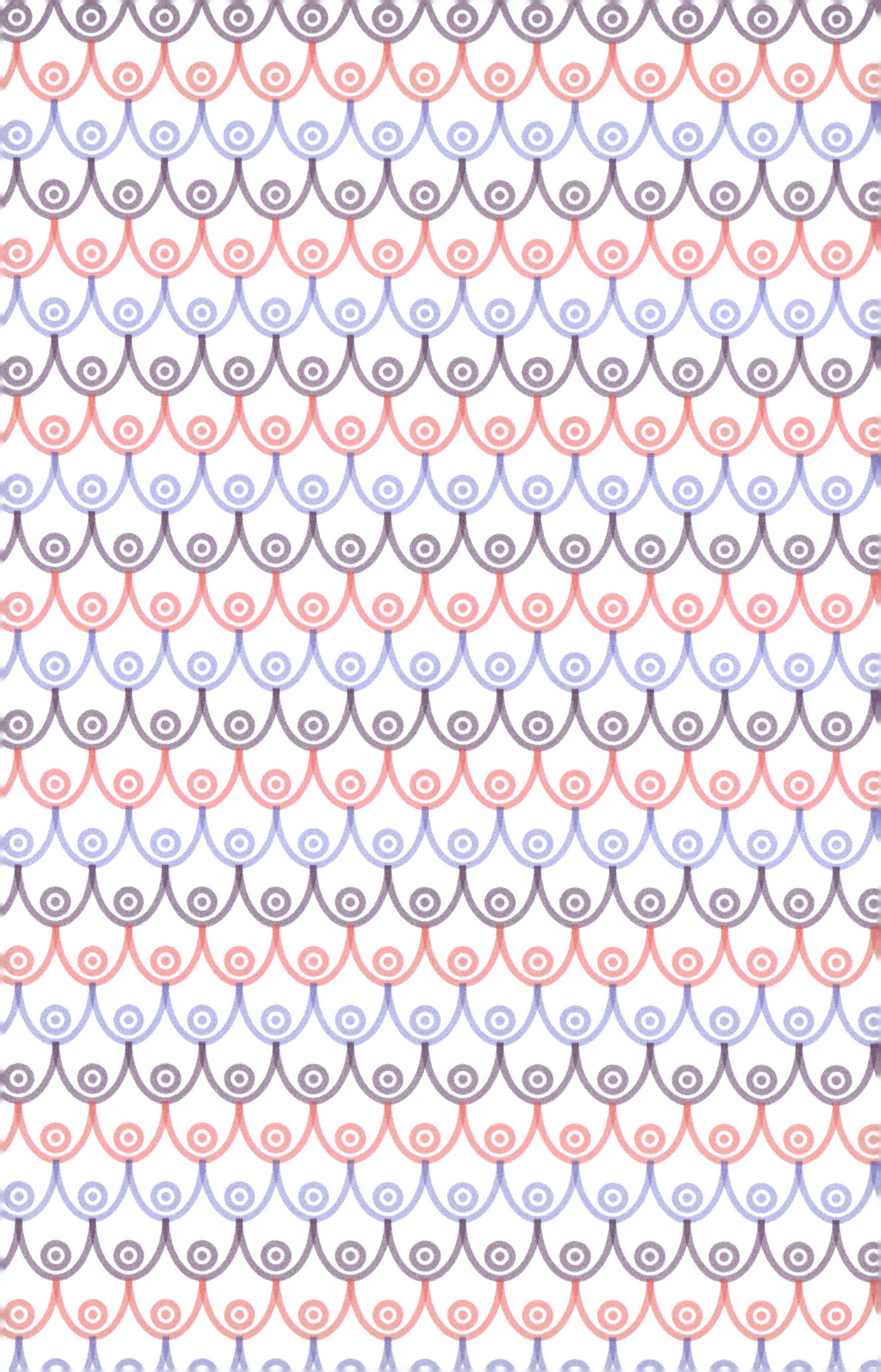

TAOISM
AND
SEXUAL QIGONG

Taoism and Dualism

Our western world image is built upon science-based thought patterns from the 17th century. It is dualistic and distinguishes between spirit and matter. Science has taught us a lot about technology, medicine, history and psychology, and how the human body is built. But it can't explain our consciousness, spirituality or what self-healing is. What we call "reality" is what can be tested and proven repeatedly with similar experiments with the same result, while we often ignore the "unreal" that can't be tested in the same way. But all insights can't be reached through the intellect. Researchers can't, at first, know what they will discover, but have to believe in their idea. Or as one of my Qigong teachers said "You don't have to understand to believe, but you must believe to understand".

Taoism is several thousand years old and has a more holistic worldview. It was developed in China, and Lao Tzu (about 400 BC) is usually regarded as its founder. The philosophical writing of Tao Te Ching, "The Classic of the Way and Virtue", is usually linked to him and perceived as a classic. It consists of a collection of philosophical and enigmatic texts that begin with the lines:

The Tao that can be observed is not the eternal Tao.
What can be named is not the eternal name.
The indescribable is the origin of the universe.

One of the most popular female practitioners of Taoism was Sun Bu'er, poet and mystic. She lived in the 1100's and gave birth to three children and began practicing single cultivation of the senses and mind when she was 51 years old and, according to the story, then went into full enlightenment. Among other things, she wrote poetry about internal alchemy for women. The poems also concern original spirit, the one that existed before our physical body came into the world, the one which does not change. What changes is the consciously embossed ego. By emptying the mind, the original spirit can take place again in our hearts.

Like many other spiritual philosophies and thought traditions, parts of Taoism can be traced back to shamanic traditional heritage. This was what one of my teachers found when searching for the roots of the Taoist practises. All shamanic cultures have similar approaches, which usually include studies of nature and its forces, and "travel" between different "worlds" or different states of consciousness, thereby finding wisdom about life, nature and the universe. Mystics have rarely been interested in religion, but more of direct experience. Knowledge must be tested before it becomes true wisdom.

Taoism and quantum physics

The Taoists were free thinkers and scientists who explored the body, but they also investigated the more difficult energy attributes of the body. They perceived everything to be energy. Reality can be investigated from two directions, as matter and as energy. It is not either or, but both. This has also brought our western science to Einstein's famous equation $E = mc2$ (energy = matter) from 1905. We have probably not fully understood the meaning of this yet, as it takes time for new thought patterns to permeate into our consciousness. Quantum physics perceives energy as both points and waves. It says that everything is a whole built out of the same small elements. All is vibrations, bioelectric energy (electromagnetism, + pole and - pole), which we can sense or feel intuitively. This has recently been able to be measured and proven with technology. Every structure in the universe, from a cell to an organ to a human to a planet, has its own unique energy pattern. A force field of electromagnetic charges and information found in and around everything, from the smallest quantum particles to celestial bodies in the cosmos. Something which Taoists and many others from different indigenous cultures understood and explored since ancient times.

In Taoism, they have investigated what we humans are and tried to understand the universe by exploring our inner worlds, which includes both the body and the soul. Everyone has a physical body and an energy body and none of them are better or worse than the other. They represent two sides of the same coin. The difference is that one is visible and the other is invisible. The same thing has been found in quantum physics. Atoms consist largely of "invisible" energy. This is also called "dark matter". The universe is not an empty void between the planets, but a dynamic unity. Many older traditions mean that the "visible" reality is a mirror of the "invisible", and that it is in the "invisible" world that the "visible" is created. Quantum physics have also stated that whenever they create something, "antimatter" is also created, the opposite of "common" matter and they are each other's reflection. This is still a mysterious and inexplicable phenomenon in science.

In many traditions, the idea is that our existence has two aspects. We can recognize the saying "on earth, as it is in heaven" from Christianity. Others speak of as above and so below, "body and soul", "energy and matter", "form and formlessness", "microcosm and macrocosm" or "yin and yang".

Yin and yang

Tao means "the path" and Taoism is more of a philosophy of life and a science than a religion. One basic assumption is that everything in the universe is forever changing. Two well-known concepts from the Taoist philosophy are yin and yang, two opposing forces sprung from Tao that represent different aspects of the whole. These energies are in constant transformation, they constantly strive for equilibrium and can not exist without each other. Everything can be described as yin or yang and everything is relative.

All people have both yin and yang within themselves. It is reflected in our brain hemispheres, where the right is more linked to creative (yin, nonlinear) thinking while the left to logical (yang, linear) thinking. Observing and focusing on energy stimulates the cognitive and linear side. To experience and feel stimulates the intuitive and nonlinear side. In order to maintain harmony within yourself and in your life, you need a balance between the creative and the logical.

> *The importance of restoring the balance between the male and female within us can not be emphasized enough.*

Female and male

The feminine and masculine are examples of two opposing forces. The female is associated with yin, a receptive creative energy with qualities like magic, intuition, being, the inner and the unknown. Already in the writing of Tao Te Ching, the woman is referred to as "the mysterious female, the gateway to the elevated". The male is yang, the active and fertilizing power associated with logic, achievement, doing, the outer and the known. A society in which logical thinking and the external are favored and the magical inner dimensions are reduced, risks becoming insensitive to the feminine, female sexuality and female mysterious. Examples of this are when soft values such as care and respect for nature and life are underestimated, and also disregarding the magic and healing ability of our own body.

An important part of the quest to restore the balance of our planet is to reaffirm and regain the feminine qualities. In general, one can say that a woman needs to start by going inwards to gain strength to become powerful. And isn't it noticeable when women - and men - missed this first step and "just" assumed authority in a more "masculine" way? A man also needs to start by going inward, to find his real purpose, then he can go out into the world and "make it". But both women and men need to get acquainted with each other's essences and we need each other to become whole. Yin and Yang are dancing with each other in a mutual eternal romance.

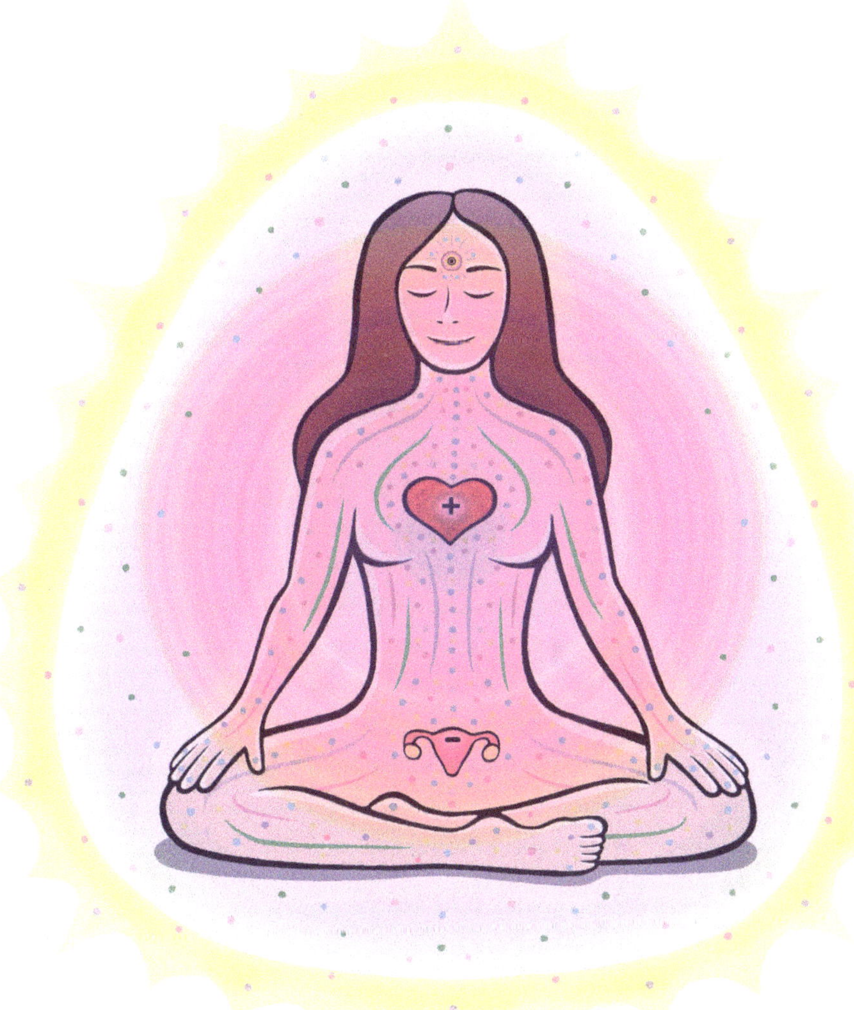

All is energy. Everything is electromagnetic fields with positive and negative charges pulsating in you. The woman is positively charged in the heart and negatively charged in the sex. For the man it is the other way around.

Another concept in Tao is that a woman is negatively (yin) charged in the genitals and positively (yang) charged in the heart while in the man it is the other way around. This means that a woman gives with her heart (love) and receives with her the genitals (sexuality) and the man gives with his genitals and receives with his heart. If we generalize, this means that the female is more focused on feelings and the male more on sex. In the best of worlds women support men to open their hearts and men support women to open up sexually. An immature expression of this is that a woman "just wants to get married" or that a man "just wants sex" without respect for the partner. A woman who unilaterally searches to be close without the ability of sexual dedication, is as half and incomplete as a man only seeking for ejaculation and orgasm, without the ability of emotional connection.

In the differences between man and woman, there is much joy and inspiration. Between these two polarities, yin and yang, flows energy, like an electromagnetic field, in ourselves as well as between men and women. These are examples of differences, but in our very innermost nature we are all the same and everything is one.

> *A woman who unilaterally searches to be close without the ability of sexual dedication, is as half and incomplete as a man only seeking for ejaculation and orgasm, without the ability of emotional connection.*

Both women and men need to see the whole picture and have full acceptance for all aspects of life. An equilibrium can then be manifested into life and help to end the collective war between patriarchy and matriarchy. Our relationships reflect us. Awareness of different aspects and a non-judgmental attitude is the key, as well as understanding that you have a choice to make a shift and that it is you that direct your energy. The practices in this book will help you better understand the existence of yin and yang within yourself and will also promote increased awareness of your thought and behavior patterns as well as your choices. In the book "Don Juan and the Art of Sexual Energy" (Tunneshende), Don Juan even believes that the most important thing you can do, and a must to restore the balance of the world, is to regain the power of the womb and reclaim your ability to orgasm.

Sex and Spirituality

Since the beginning of time, humanity has been fascinated by the sexual power, which ensures our survival and thus "immortality." In China, it was discovered a long time ago, that the key to a long life of happiness and health lies in the cultivation of the sexual essence. From this wisdom Taoist sexual Qigong was created. Sexual essence signify reproduction and production of sex hormones as well as our desire for pleasure and creational potential. Tao further says that; *If you can not meet your sexuality directly, you will never discover your true spirituality. To understand what will make you "immortal", study what created you.*

The power of God, fertility and the games of love has always been interconnected. Most thought traditions have also had different ways of managing or regulating the sexual energy. Ranging from sexual abstinence and joining monasteries, circulating divine energy in Tantra (a philosophy and practical spiritual science with roots in India), exploring different aspects of your personality in the shamanic love art Quodoushka ("the twisted hairs elders", a tradition from the American continents) to various ancient fertility rituals. And considering how many religions perceive erotic pleasure, there seems to be something that is either dangerous and threatening, or special and magical. Sex and spirit seem to belong together. In the collection of essays, "Sex – för guds skull (Sex – for God's Sake)" they even asked "religion and sex, how can they be separated?" The texts deal with sexuality and eroticism in the major world religions and how they judge what is good or bad sexuality.

In the traditions of Tao, Tantra and Quodoushka, they consider the sexual act as a meeting, a creative force, an exchange of energy or the union of sexuality and spirituality (yin and yang, body and soul, earth and sky, matter and energy) and the result is larger than the parts. This meeting happens all the time in nature, for example when the bee pollinates the flower, when the seed of an apple finds its place in the ground or even when the rays of the sun provide energy that the soil receives. Sexuality and spirituality do not stand in contrast to each other, but on the contrary, one cannot exist without the other.

So what is sexual Qigong and what can it do for you?

Qi, Qigong and Chinese medicine

Qigong is a collective name for thousands of different types of practices and meditations. The name came about around 200 BC, according to one of my Qigong teachers, when different tribes in China gathered to share their practice and knowledge. The wisdom is founded on thousands of years of experience and is sometimes called Taoist Yoga (yoga is sanskrit and means union). The Qigong styles have different Chinese names. I teach, for example, Xing Shen Zhuang, Tao Yin and Wuji Gong. There are Taoist, Buddhist and Tibetan Qigong. Qigong exercises often affect several aspects of us, but may have a slightly different orientation, such as mental, emotional, physical, spiritual or sexual. They can be performed sitting, lying or standing, and are usually in the form of slow soft movements. Something that all of them have in common is the importance of good posture, relaxation and inner focus for the purpose of promoting well-being. Today, it is common to practice medical Qigong which focuses on better health, but from the beginning, the practice of Qigong was also a spiritual path, as it still is today for many practitioners.

Qi means "life force" and gong means "practice". Qigong is thus a way to train and cultivate your life force energy. The term Qi is found in several cultures and has been found in many other languages, such as prana (Indian), lung (Tibetan), ruach (Hebrew), num (Kalahari), chuluaqui (Cherokee) and ki (Japanese) to name a few. Good health is the same as a harmonious flow of Qi in the body's meridians (energy channels). All Taoist Qigong exercises are about strengthening and balancing Qi in various ways.

Qi can be compared to what we call bioelectric energy. Research has been able to show that every cell in our body, and even the entire universe, consists of energy and electrical charges. Each electrical impulse creates a surrounding electromagnetic force field. Qi assumes different forms and is described in terms of various quality, strength and quantity. Qi is constantly flowing through your body. Everything from a rock to a tree to the whole universe has its own kind of Qi and you also have your own Qi, which makes you unique.

Qi circulates through the body along the meridians, on which the acupuncture points are located. By reading the pulse in the meridians, an acupuncturist can alert you of imbalances before they do any excessive damage. There are twelve primary meridians connected to different internal organs and eight other channels, of which we will explore three: Du Mai (going up the spine), Ren Mai (down the front of your body) and Chong Mai (a channel thrusting through the middle of the body). Traditional Chinese Medicine (TCM) includes, in addition to acupuncture: herbs, Qigong, massage as well as astrology and Feng Shui.

In TCM, the "five element theory" is used to diagnose and describe symptoms and conditions. Fire, earth, metal, water and wood represent different aspects and characteristics within us and are also associated with different internal organs. Tao believes that all aspects of life can be reflected in the elements. Read more about the elements and their connections to emotions, organs and more on page 99.

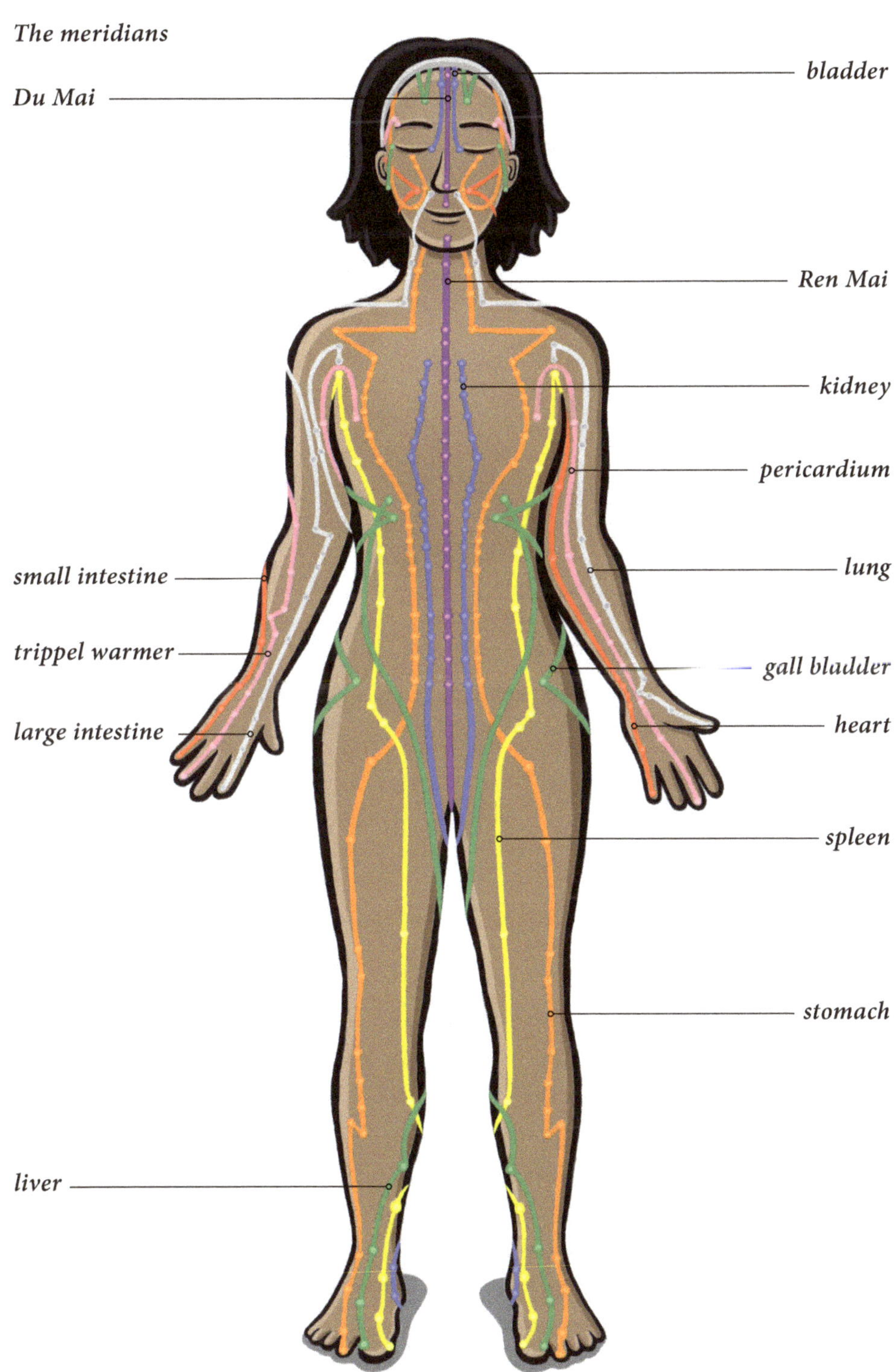

Qi is circulated through your body along energy paths, called meridians, connected to different organs.

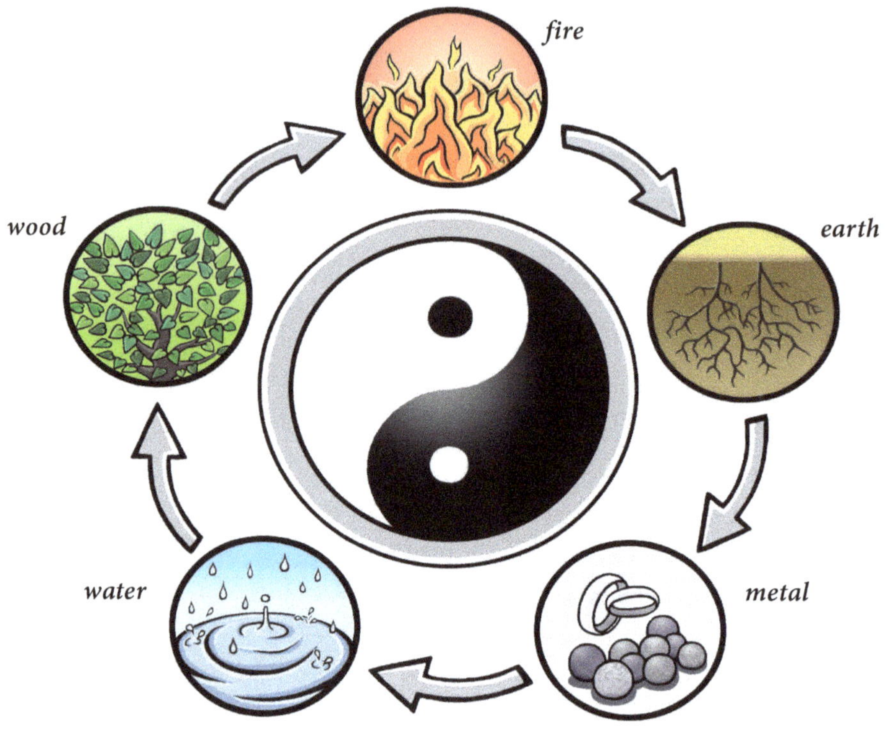

Sexual energy

Various thought traditions describe the erotic potential as something special. In the Indian tantric tradition, this slumbering power is seen as cosmic energy and symbolically depicted as a snake awakening and traveling up the spine. Therefore, it is called kundalini (Sanskrit for coiled). In the shamanic tradition, sexuality is represented as our natural right to be ecstatic; it is our creative life force, where the birthing of physical children is only one possibility of many. In Taoism, sexuality is our capacity for optimal health and life experience. Tao even views it as a way to be able to slow down the aging process. In other contemporary religions it is instead associated with shame and guilt while those who live beyond sexuality and marriage are elevated.

Getting conscious access to, and cultivating, your sexual energy is the foundation of this Taoistic training. The exercises teach you how to guide the energy into your body instead of projecting it outward. By doing so, you gain access to your life energy which can improve your well-being and enhance your life experience. If you had full integrity in your sexual drive it would probably be a revolution in your way of creating relationships. Try to imagine how you would choose a partner if the attraction was not controlled by more or less unsatisfied unconscious erotic desires and emotional needs. It doesn't mean that the desire is not there, it's only more intentional and closer to your true desire and needs of your heart.

The role that sexual energy plays in the Taoist practices here is probably different and perhaps far from how you are used to thinking about and relating to this type of energy. It doesn't have much to do with sexuality as we are used to perceiving it. Thus, not a twosome relegated to a bedroom, in the worst case, only to have an outlet of frustration or an indefinite longing. Instead, it is perceived as a neutral energy, a creative potential whose intelligence can support your practice and your life in every possible fruitful way. Sexual energy is objective and neither good nor bad. Different values and moral condemnations rather come from different cultural and religious imprints.

> *If you had full integrity in your sexual drive, it would probably be a revolution in your way of creating relationships.*

Is it possible to liberate your sexual power from your personal and cultural values? A first step is to perceive it in a new way and free it from emotions and dependencies that prevent us from expressing ourselves naturally as women. Instead, see it as a gift, a power that we have access to and which manifests in the body. It is common for us to burden our sexuality with shame and guilt. Instead, let it be, regardless of your story, just as it is, without judging your sexual power from right or wrong. Not as an uncontrolled drive but with integrity and respect for all life. You can't change your past but you can always change your attitude and, by doing so, transform the moment in a blink of an eye. Allow yourself to look at yourself with new eyes. Try the exercise on page 97 on the intelligence of the heart.

A catalyzing force

The sexual energy is our strongest and most powerful energy. It is a catalytic force that amplifies everything, like $1 + 1 = 3$, or the baking soda in your cake. If you skip the baking soda, the result will be a rather bland and flat sponge cake. The sexual energy strengthens what is already there. Keep in mind that this applies to all kinds of emotions. The orgasmic potency is strongly linked to creational power, actualization and materialization of desires and dreams. The same power that literally has the potential to create new life, you can also use for your self-realization.

Sexual Qigong in theory

All of us are born with a certain potential characterized by the union between our parents and their genealogy. It gave us a certain amount of foundational life energy. This innate energy is called Jing and represents our essence. Jing is the energy behind our drive to reproduce and our desire to use our creational power. It is the fuel for sexuality, hormone production and menstrual cycle. Our heritage is complemented by the energy we obtain from the air we breathe and the food we eat. We also gain power from being in nature, exercising, resting or sleeping. Everything is included in the term Jing.

Then you make use of the energy through, for example, work, digestion and metabolism and various activities. As the years go by and depending on your lifestyle, you start overtaxing your energy resources and relinquishing the reserves, which, within TCM in particular, is associated with the kidneys and your essence. Your vital organs, such as kidneys, spleen, lungs, liver and heart, then glands and eventually the brain, become overburdened. You start consuming more than you add or can absorb and aging accelerates.

> *Jing, the sexual energy, is a force that seems infinite and it is also the only force that can be doubled.*

According to the Taoists, it is a very energy-demanding process for the body to produce sperm and eggs. Women lose mainly their vitality through heavy menstruations (blood and egg) and man through ejaculation (sperm). Therefore, the exercises in this book are also designed to reduce these processes, which is why they are different for women and men.

At the same time you have an abundance of innate energy. Jing, the sexual energy, is a force that seems infinite and it is also the only force that can be doubled. For many of us, the mere thought of it is literally enough to speed up our sexual flow. It is this Jing force that we use, recycle and refine in sexual Qigong. Raw sexual energy becomes nutrition for body and soul.

Sexual alchemy

Symbolically, the Taoists perceive the sexual energy as water (a sea of possibilities) and the heart as fire (the soul, thoughts and feelings). If you do not master the fire, its energy simply goes up in smoke. For example, to ponder or get lost in emotional dramas are processes that burn a lot of energy. The water, in turn, flows down and away unless you reverse the flow, which you do when learning to guide your sexual energy up the spine.

Sexual alchemy can be equated to the sun shining on a lake. The heat warms the water, which turns into steam rising up and that then rains down to give life and nutrition. Kan (water) and Li (fire) are the Taoist names of these processes. It's when we change the direction of these flows that we can reverse the aging process.

Alchemy means "the study of refinement" and is founded on the assumption that everything is connected and that all subjects actually come from one source. By distinguishing and directing a substance back to the source it can become purified, transformed and even given completely new features. Taoism is filled with internal alchemy where, among other things, the elements (fire, earth, metal, water and wood) represent different characteristics that are intertwined in various ways within us to achieve different states. If we translate the symbolism above into your life, it becomes an essential task, to combine your sexuality with your heart and love. Or, the reverse, to pair up the love with eroticism. In the following exercises, you practice reversing the orgasmic flow of life and balancing your emotions. You create integrity both in your feelings and in your sexuality as well as the feeling of being whole and embracing a passionate self-love. A natural ability to impregnate yourself with the desire of your heart and your highest potential.

> *In Taoism, sexuality is our capacity for optimal health and life experience.*

You can learn how to convert your sexual power as well as energy from food, air and your environment into Qi, life energy, which supplies the organs of the body with the necessary energy. This energy can then be transformed into Shen, awareness or spiritual energy, which in turn is reunited with the "void" or original spirit and its potential. In Qigong we describe our vitality on the basis of these three concepts - Jing, Qi and Shen.

I will continue to use different names for Jing, such as sexual energy, essence, catalytic force, erotic potential, libido etc. with the hope that you keep its broader significance in mind.

The three treasures

If you ask Westerners what the purpose of Qigong is, they would probably respond with "improving health" or "preventing ill health". If you asked a Tao master, they would probably answer "to unite the three treasures of life energy, Jing, Qi and Shen". Taoist wisdom and theory are very rich and not always easy to explain, but generally, and very simplified, the purpose of the practice is to transform sexual energy into life energy and, in turn, to expand consciousness. That's what is called the three treasures (The Taoist name is San Bao). Transformation occurs in different ways and places in the body. Three important places are the three Dan Tian (elixir fields). If the meridians are like rivers in the body where energy can flow, these are lakes where energy can be gathered. Lower Dan Tian, an area in the lower abdomen behind and below the navel will be the most important for these exercises. There is also middle Dan Tian, behind the sternum, in the heart center and upper Dan Tian behind the 3rd eye, in the middle of the forehead slightly into the head.

The three treasures of life energy:

Jing = Our original energy, the sexual power, erotic fluids, hormones and reproduction ability. Linked to our heritage, DNA. Also described as essence. Associated with the physical body and the kidneys. Here is the fuel.

Qi = Life force, life energy, vitality. Associated with your energy body and all kinds of motion, breathing and circulation. If Jing is the fuel in the power plant, this is the electricity.

Shen = Spiritual energy, consciousness, the soul that is reflected in the eyes. Associated with wisdom, compassion and enlightenment. This is the light which radiates from the electricity.

Dan Tian

Lower Dan Tian is an important place in all exercises. Several spiritual paths and martial arts talk about the importance of the connection to your center. It is located in the lower abdomen, behind and below the navel. It is a space inside, a sphere. It's a neutral place where you can ground your experiences and gather all the energy you create. The more centered you are, the less the outside can affect you. If you keep your center, you can be yourself and your energy can remain in harmony and balance. By consciously focusing your breath and attention to this place, energy can accumulate and develop. This is where you can store energy to "charge the batteries". I supplies energy to the meridian system. Compare it to depositing Qi into your energy account, to be used as

The three Dan Tian

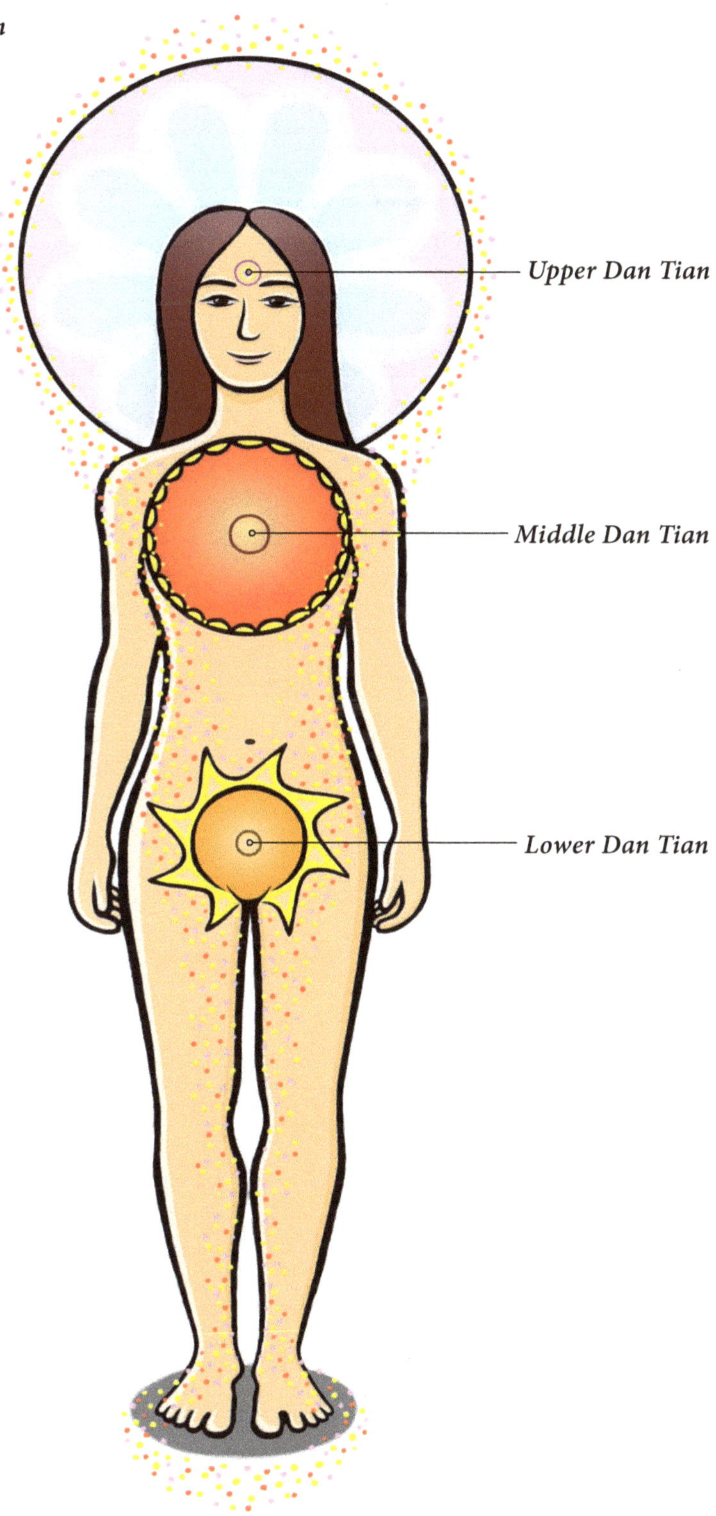
Upper Dan Tian
Middle Dan Tian
Lower Dan Tian

needed. Lower Dan Tian is good at storing energy, while for example the brain is good at receiving energy and the genitals are good at generating energy.

This "brain" of Dan Tian, is what Western medicine calls the "abdominal brain" or the enteric nervous system, which, through its many linking nerves, basically has the same ability of consciousness as our "normal" brain. It is also here that you can cultivate your observational ability and your connection to that which never changes in you, that which is always whole.

> *It is also here that you can cultivate your observational ability and your connection to that which never changes in you, that which is always whole.*

Your own Dan Tian, however, is not something you can take for granted, but is something you are a co-creator of throughout life. It is your potential which you can manage well by regularly giving nutrition and attention to its fertile ground. Within Tao, it is seen as a spiritual conception where your so-called spiritual child can begin to be brought to life. The Taoists imagine spiritual conception as an imitation of physical conception. They are a reflection of each other. Creational power is the most powerful energy we have. To nurture Dan Tian, is also an internal practice to awaken the potential of your womb space.

Henceforth, the lower Dan Tian in the lower abdomen, will be called Dan Tian.

The kidneys, the batteries of the body

In Chinese medicine, the kidneys are the root of the original spirit and are linked to the Dan Tian. The center of the kidneys, between the lumbar vertebrae 2 and 3, is called Ming Men which means the "Gate of Life". They hold the wisdom of the body and our heritage. The kidneys can be seen as the batteries of our body. If kept well and healthy, they can support all the other organs. They can be charged or discharged. Stress, anxiety and an unfavorable lifestyle can easily deplete your batteries. When caught up mainly in the external and losing your center, you create fear and stress. The kidneys are connected intimately to your sexual energy and creative power. It is the adrenal glands that especially store your legacy and your basic vitality. In Western medicine it has been found that the ovaries in the fetus are formed from the kidneys. It is also known that healthy ovaries have difficulties functioning if the adrenal glands are injured or depleted, while inferior ovaries function fine as long as the adrenal glands are healthy.

FOUNDATIONAL PRINCIPLES

Grounding

Grounding is about presence and being aware of your thoughts, feelings, bodily sensations, intentions and the whole life experience. The more grounded you are in yourself and your body, the easier it is to get through strong emotional experiences in life. With a stable body you can allow your emotions to flow through without losing yourself. Your awareness and your mind can be trained to embrace and hold all the sensations in the body. Your mind is not concentrated in your head, it is distributed throughout the body through the nervous system. You can trust that your nervous system is organized to take care of you.

> *The more grounded you are in yourself and your body, the easier it is to get through strong emotional experiences in life.*

Being able to stay within a feeling, allowing it to pass and accept it has a strong healing and transforming effect. Emotions seem to be meant to flow through the body, they are things that come and go naturally. Being able to listen to your body's signals is an ability you can train through increased bodily awareness. There is a saying that goes: "If you can hear your body whisper, you don't need to hear it scream". Qigong focuses a great deal on this. This awareness makes it easier for you to feel and thus act based on your real needs and resist the countless temptations which you are constantly exposed to in your daily life.

As you learn how to recognize the signals of your body, you also become more aware of both your thoughts and feelings and the relationships between them. You can distinguish emotions that are just a response to past reactions and get their fuel from past situations, from those which are more about instincts and an inner knowing of what's right.

In these exercises, we always start turning the focus inward and then we finish all exercises in the lower Dan Tian. We gather the energy and ground ourselves there. It is the core of the body, where you have your center of gravity and can anchor yourself. You are grounding yourself in your body, and it in turn needs to be grounded in the earth.

Earthing

Grounding is also about contact with Mother Earth. By connecting to it through your feet, especially through the 1st meridian point of the kidney, you can connect with the ground. Kidney 1 is called "gushing spring" and sits in the middle of the foot just behind the front foot pad. As we have seen before, all is electrical charges. Radiation from our environment, both natural and unnatural, unfavorable food and stress lead to a surplus of positive ions (atoms and molecules), which creates deteriorating processes in the body. Earth is charged with negative ions. Studies has shown that the Earth's surplus of negative ions can balance our bodies, which, for example, positively affect our immune system. By walking barefoot in nature you can balance the ions of the body and thus create greater equilibrium in your cells and vital systems. Earthing leads to relaxation, better sleep and new power. Feel free to practice Qigong outdoors and barefoot when you can.

Good posture is like Feng Shui for the body

After 20 years of daily training, one of my Qigong teachers announced that he had finally learned to stand correctly and that he could now also sit quite well. While he was talking about the lotus position, this still shows that we can all improve our body posture. To stand still in different positions is a whole school within Qigong and which we will practice through an exercise called the tree. There is a great need in our society for education on posture and movement patterns. Many of us have had back problems and many of us will. As much as 70% of all back problems are believed to be due to unfavorable posture. If you look around, it's easy to find that some people tend to stand, walk and sit with a curved back, sunken upper body and a vulture neck. It also adversely affects the breathing and Qi flow. It, in turn, unfavorably affects the oxygenation of the blood, which leads to ... Yes, as you can see, a negative spiral has been triggered - the it goes on and on.

From merely a slight imbalance in your body, or from maybe sitting somewhat crooked, a muscle can be forced to work constantly to maintain equilibrium. An important muscle, which is often involved in different types of back pain, is psoas, the hip flexor. The Taoists call it the "muscle of the soul" and it is important for our grounding and connection between upper and lower body as well as with the earth and our life experience.

With a good balance in your posture you will be as steady as a tree and your muscles will be relieved. They only need to work a minimum, otherwise they can relax and rest. Muscles certainly like and need training, but not static or obliquely. Because then they get tense over time and start to hurt.

The tendons attach the muscles to the skeleton and it is very important that they are kept agile. If you do not stretch, they become brittle and stiff and can easily rip, just like a dry old rubber band that lost its elasticity. The tendons, like the connective tissue and fascia, are significant conductors of Qi. The muscles need relaxation, the tendons and fascia need stretching and slow motion, then the joints and connective tissue will be softened up. Changing an incorrect posture requires conscious pursuit for quite some time.

In Qigong we work a great deal on correcting bad bodily habits and becoming aware of tension. It's like Feng Shui for your body where the goal for the energy is to dance as freely and naturally as possible. Feng Shui means "wind and water" and teaches how energy can flow and function best in a given place. In this case, your body. The body wants to be illuminated by your consciousness. Keep in mind the claim that "all ails begin with poor circulation", for your motivation to increase further. That idea was pronounced by Huang-Di, also known as "The Yellow Emperor" (about 2,600 BC), who is said to be a co-creator of the Chinese classical medical work Huang Di Nei Jing, "The Inner Canon of the Yellow Emperor".

With a good balance in your posture you will be as steady as a tree and your muscles will be relieved.

The breath is the bridge between body and soul

Breathing acts as a bridge between consciousness and the physical. Through the breath you can connect to your inner world, guide your consciousness inward and direct it to different parts of your body. The breath raises awareness in the cells. When the lungs are filled with air, they supply the blood with oxygen, which is an important function for giving the cells energy and ability for renewal. Equally important is the exhalation where carbon dioxide, a residual product from metabolism and cellular respiration, leaves the body. The Taoists call the diaphragm the "muscle of the spirit", with which it is important to have a connection. The word Qigong can also be interpreted as processing and refining breathing. So be sure to breathe deeply and sometimes completely empty your lungs. By doing so the life force enters and with a strong exhale you are then pushing out waste products. Breathing is one of our most important aids for cleaning the body of waste products.

Circulation, blood and consciousness

The Yellow Emperor's thought "where there is good circulation there are no ails, poor circulation leads to pain" is interesting. He meant that unfavorable circulation is the basis of all disease because poison accumulates and acidifies the tissues of the body. Blood circulation is essential for the transportation of oxygen, nutrition and hormones to cells as well as for disposing of waste through exhalation, sweat, urine and stool.

Tao also states that the blood, through the breath, is a carrier of consciousness into the body. The heart pumping the blood symbolizes your innermost and your capacity to unite with the spirit. Imagine the importance that every time you breathe in, you fill, through the oxygen and your blood, every cell of consciousness, with all that you are, your stories, your values, your attitude and your purpose created in that moment. And when you breathe out, you share this with the outside world.

Muscles of the soul and spirit

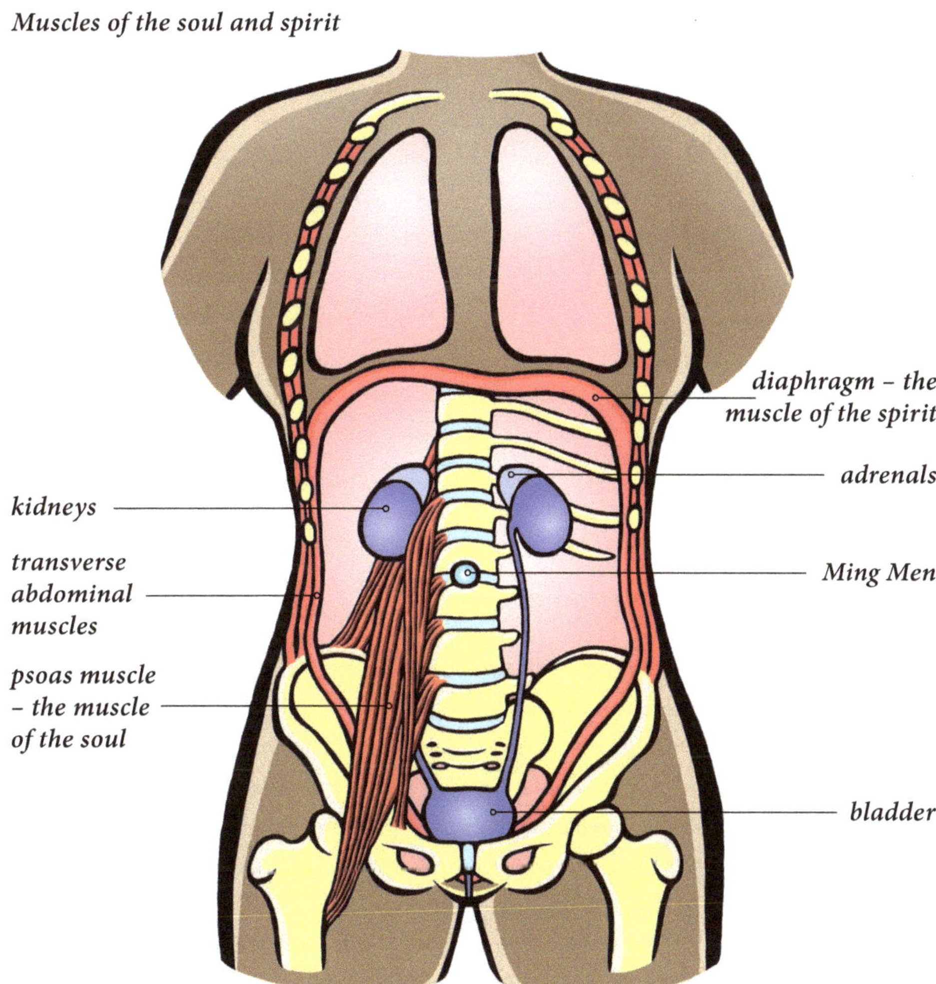

The condition of the psoas, diaphragm and kidneys is intimately connected and is important for our well-being. The kidneys are the "batteries" of your body. If kept well, including tissues around, they can help support all other organs.

The nervous system

The central nervous system (CNS) consists of the brain, brainstem and spinal cord and communicates with and directs all parts of the body. The peripheral nervous system (PNS) is usually divided into two parts, the somatic (will-ruled) and the autonomous (non-willed). The autonomic nervous system manages the regulation of cardiac activity, blood circulation, digestion, gland operations and other activities that we can't control with our will. Most often, the enteric nervous system (ENS, lower abdominal brain) is also included in the autonomous part, and is a system that manages the gastrointestinal tract functions. However, because it contains more nerve cells than the spinal cord and can function without any contact with the CNS, it is increasingly regarded as one of the three major components of the nervous system.

> *The endocrine glands and hormone system are fundamental to your cycles and your well-being.*

The autonomous part of the nervous system is divided into two parts, the sympathetic and the parasympathetic nervous system. When the sympathetic nervous system is activated, the body is ready to act or to run or defend itself, which causes heart rate and blood pressure to increase. The muscles get ready and the internal systems such as digestion have less access to energy. When you are at risk, it is more important to prepare for escape than to digest your food. When activating the parasympathetic nervous system, adverse effects are observed. Heart activity decreases, blood pressure decreases and digestion is stimulated. You feel calm and relaxed.

Hormones, how do they know what to do?

The nervous system and the hormone system are the most important communication systems in our body. The endocrine glands secrete hormones, small information carriers that are transported in the body by the blood, usually in proteins or fat cells. Some hormones are called neurotransmitters and are then transmitted primarily through nerve connections. If you compare the body to a company, the hypothalamus (which is both an endocrine gland and part of the nervous system) in the brain, is the board and the pituitary gland is the CEO that initiates the processes while the hormones perform the actual work. The endocrine glands and hormone system are fundamental to your cycles and your well-being. Today, it is not uncommon to have imbalances in the thyroid gland. About ten percent of all women in Sweden are predisposed to have an underactive or overactive thyroid gland. This contributes, among other things, to reduced energy levels and fatigue. Lack of equilibrium in the hormone system also appears as PMS (premenstrual syndrome) and menopause problems as well as stress-related symptoms.

Understanding how hormones work on a deeper level is not easy. It is a highly complex system that is basically involved in all processes in the body and there is still an endless amount of things to discover in this area. The research is complicated by the fact that the chemical messengers often work together, which increases the difficulty of seeing the whole picture when they are studied separately. Many researchers are fascinated by the question of how the hormones actually know what to do. Does the cell have a consciousness? In Taoist theory, hormones are seen as part of your essence and are included in the term Jing. They keep track of the information and are the key to different processes in the body. It's like the chemical messengers know when it's time for different things. They have a clear intention, but are also affected by the environment. In the chapter on menopause (p. 80) and and in the exercise hormone shower (p. 118) you can read more about glands and hormones.

Cell renewal

The cells are the most important building blocks of the body. Our body is made up of cells that, in turn, form fluids, tissues and organs. A person consists of about 50 trillion cells! Every day, several billions of cells die in your body and new ones are created all the time. Different types of cells have different lifespans. The lifetime of a skin cell is 28 days, the mucous membrane of the intestine is renewed after 72 hours, while the bone marrow needs the longest time to regenerate; about 7 years. We depend on our breath to get rid of the carbon dioxide from dead cells and provide living cells with fresh oxygen. This process is vital for our survival. In order to produce healthy cells, we also need hydrogen, carbon and other minerals and vitamins which we absorb from food. The cell is like a small factory, or its own individual, who wants the best raw material (nutrients), a supportive environment (acid-base balance, ph-value), appreciation (attitude) and clear directives (hormones, intent). In short, the cell is much like you and me.

The quality of the air, the purity of the water, the choice of food, good physique and nourishing thoughts are important in terms of good health and a long life. The cell is dependent on sleep, which is when most renewal occurs. It is also influenced by our experiences. It is the bearer of our heritage and has a cell memory back from several generations. Each new cell allows you to program a healing and strengthening attitude and new inspirational intentions. This way you can break destructive patterns and support the self-healing ability of your body and reunite with your deepest loving nature.

Cell consciousness

A question that researchers have discussed for a long time is whether we are governed most by heritage or environment. Research on the cell in recent years has shown that the environment affects the behavior of the cell without changing the genetic code. Experiments have repeatedly shown how important the environment is, for example, to develop a negative heritage or not. The cell can analyze thousands of stimuli from the environment it is in. The cells of our nervous system are experts in reading the environment through our minds and senses.

Our conscious mind is superior to all.

This means that we are not victims of our genes, but we in many ways control our destiny. A gene can not switch itself on or off, that impulse or intelligence comes from the outside world. In his interesting and clarifying book "The Biology of Belief", Bruce H. Lipton even says that the cells not only teach us about the mechanics of life, but they also show us how to live a rich and full life. He believes that it is not our hormones and neurotransmitters that control the body and the functions of our minds with the help of genes, but that it is our convictions and beliefs that control everything. Our conscious mind is superior to all.

Values, attitude and focus

There is a saying that claims that everything is about your attitude. Your attitude determines how you view different things in life and your ability to accept new ideas and thoughts. You can not change your history but you can change both yourself and your attitude. The thoughts, feelings and sensations you feed yourself are as important as what you put in your mouth. One of the most important things you can do in life is to become aware of your thoughts and the reality they create and learn how to choose other thoughts. Your greatest enemy hides inside your own head.

Do you believe in yourself? The American car manufacturer Henry Ford once said, "Whether you think you can, or think you can't, you're right". What do you choose to believe in? What thoughts do you fill your mind or consciousness with? Are these attitudes, belief systems, and faiths which favors and support you, or oppose you? Are these strategies that work? A Taoist saying goes: "Life is simple, we are the ones creating problems".

It's easy to change or create a feeling or a mood. Goodwill or a thought is usually enough. The challenge lies in creating a long-term sustainable attitude. A stable attitude that is in accordance with your heart's desire and purpose.

Your attitude, and above all, the ability to focus your attention in the desired direction is important for your success in the exercises. By focusing on a part of your body, it causes increased activity in the nerves, muscles and fascia, as well as increased blood and lymph flow. Based on Chinese medical understanding, all bodily systems are operated through Qi, which include both energy and information. Your increased concentration changes the flow of Qi, which then affects your blood flow. The clearer the focus, the more flow and more Qi will be moved to the area. Awareness about this is the basis for these practices. That energy follows thought is a reliable concept.

Purpose and intention

For an intent or intention to have power, it needs to be in harmony with all of you. In addition, it should have a motivation and your permission as well as be authenticated and grounded in your body and your feelings. All strong intentions come from the heart. They can't simply be imagined in your head, then your intention is only half-hearted. It is your will, your curiosity and the desire of your heart which determines the direction of your life. Without intention there is no direction. In Taoist philosophy there is a concept that includes intention, which implies that "intention guides Qi to produce healing". Each of us must find his or her own motivation and higher purpose that inspires us. The same goes for the exercises. What is important to you? And why is it important? When you know why, then how doesn't matter as much, as Descartes (French philosopher) is said to have taught at one point. Once you find your true motivation, the how becomes easy. In Qigong, you use your intent rather than forcing the energy with strength. All exercises in this book are created to strengthen and refine the ability of intent. Eventually, you can let go of technique and guide energy only by concentrating.

All strong intentions come from the heart. They can't simply be imagined in your head, then your intention is only half-hearted.

Placebo effect

A well-known speaker and former doctor asked his audience how many believed they could think themselves sick and almost everybody raised their hands. Then he asked how many people thought they could think themselves healthy. Almost nobody raised their hand. If the conclusion is that a person consciously or unconsciously can negatively affect their own body function by only using their own will, they should also be able to influence it positively. School medicine has found it to be time to take the placebo or the expectation effect seriously, but despite the fact that there are several scientific pilot studies showing its positive effects, they have not been followed up particularly well.

For centuries, we have relied on our expectations because there were not as many active methods as there are now, and we also emphasized on the meeting with the doctor, whose task was, among other things, to bring hope. Doctor Pehr Gustaf Cederschiöld (1782-1848) said: *Through the thought one should be able to lead, as well as bring together the vitality, to the part of the body which one pleases, and as this thought is accompanied by fear or hope, thereby contributing to cause or cure diseases.*

In the past few decades, methodological studies have shown how important the trust in the one who performs the treatment and trust in the method is, and the greater the confidence the greater the self-healing effect. Thus exists a clear link between mental attitude and bodily well-being. Bodily awareness, body perception and expected experience are closely linked.

In addition, it has been perceived that the psyche can create measurable physiological changes. Researchers have come to the conclusion that some form of dialogue between body and mind must exist for placebo to occur. Bodily awareness, body perception and expected experience are closely linked. The more you understand about this connection, the better you can understand yourself and how you can influence different states, possible imbalances and unhealthy problems.

| *When the mind changes, our entire biology is affected.*

A very unexpected outcome for doctors was a study evaluating surgery on patients with severe knee pains. They "knew" that knee surgery worked and that placebo could hardly be used within surgery. Three groups were investigated, one of whom was undergoing a fake operation while the knees of the two other groups were flushed or scraped. Both methods are common treatments of inflamed knees. All three groups were administered the same care after the procedure. The doctors were surprised that the placebo group experienced the same improvement as those who were operated upon. A placebo patient who could hardly walk earlier could now even start exercising.

In people with incurable diseases, who have lived many years longer than expected, qualities which were recognized were authenticity and insight into what was important in life. Something else that was also noticed was a sense of freedom and ability to influence their situation, as well as acceptance and a joyful experience of life. Several were also involved in various self-help activities at an early stage. Another thing that has been established to affect placebo is relaxation and a positive attitude. Stress and anxiety make the impact more difficult. So your will, faith, expectation, acceptance and bodily awareness all play an important role in what you create in your life. Nowadays, it is both tested and proven that when the mind changes, our entire biology is affected.

Meditation, witness what is

Taoist meditation can mean different things, ranging from focusing on your breathing to something similar to guided meditations or internal alchemy. The word meditation has roots in the Greek word "media histemi", meaning "being, or standing in the middle", getting back to the center and returning to silence. Where then is the center, and the center of what? According to the Taoists, the center is "that which remains", which always is and does not change. They sometimes call it Shen. Shen is not quite as easy to translate, but means "consciousness" or "soul" and also refers to the "great consciousness" or source of origin. You are not a mind living in a head but a body in the great consciousness.

When you practice these exercises with your physical body and with your energy body in the form of thoughts, emotions, life energy and sensations, you are constantly exercising your consciousness. You cultivate your ability to witness, to distance yourself, and to see the whole from a wider perspective. The effect is that you can easily guide yourself without getting mentally stuck in sensations, patterns and dramas. You are no longer dependent on maintaining a specific feeling to feel good. Well-being, instead, gains new meaning and becomes more grounded in your consciousness and witnessing what is. Our ability to self-reflect makes our minds very powerful. You can develop your consciousness in what direction you want and to what level you desire.

Interview:

The meaning of life according to Professor Wang

Wang Ting Jun (1956-2009), from northern China, was a very popular and experienced Qigong teacher who was invited to Sweden by the Qigong Institute. When asked the question on why he started practicing Qigong he replied:

When I was about 30 years old, I had a dilemma, I started asking myself: Why do I live? What is the truth about life? Therefore, I began to study philosophy. Based on the studies on traditional Chinese philosophy, I began to understand that different issues come from different levels of consciousness. That is, different states of awareness create different issues, which create different questions. And when we determine the answers, we must therefore be observant of our conscious state at the moment.

What is the meaning of life and what happens when we die? A scientist might say that death occurs when the heart stops beating, when we cease breathing, the brain stops functioning and consciousness ends, etc. But that's not what I believe. By comparison, one can take an artist. He has a completely different awareness and way of seeing things than a researcher. Therefore, they may have difficulties communicating with and understanding each other.

That means we have different states of awareness and I can sense the variations of my own state of mind. This determines how I view my situation and how I look at different things in life. If you live on the basis of the researcher's approach, death means one thing and from the artist's point of view something else.

Incorporating an approach to consciousness based on traditional Chinese philosophy called Yuan Shen gives you a completely different view. Yuan Shen means "original consciousness, the soul we were born with." In which you don't die. The same approach is also found in India. This far, I have confirmed one thing; there is no aging. Our consciousness is the same, whether we are young or old, and probably even after we die.

The consciousness doesn't disappear

When I examined Chinese philosophy and asked these deep questions, I saw that many great masters have verified and experienced the same in their search for the truth about life and death.

The exploration means that we must turn our attention inwards to get to know ourselves. The modern man is usually completely focused on the outer world and has learned a lot about managing and explaining different phenomena. But a master studies his inner world through which one learns how to feel and understand both body and soul.

This requires a special practice. Qigong in China and Yoga in India are different techniques to turn the consciousness and attention from the outer world towards focusing on the inner one, bringing it back into ourselves. To cultivate your consciousness means to increase your knowledge and to embrace more of ourselves. This also leads to a greater understanding of the outside world and the universe. Most world views believe in the thesis "as above so below".

The modern man is usually trained to try and understand the outer world but not the inner. The exercises then are often only physical gymnastic exercises. It was the searching for answers to my questions about life and death that led me to study traditional Chinese philosophy and to start practicing Qigong. I really want answers to these questions, about life and about death. And to learn how to influence our consciousness at different higher levels.

Here in the West, many seek God outside of themselves, or they may have an idea of a God who can save them, or a spirit that can perform miracles. In Chinese philosophy there is no outer god as a mediator of truth. Instead, we ourselves practice our own consciousness and try to reach a new level in order to gain new approaches and knowledge. In China, it is believed that the spirit is in all of us. We can enlighten ourselves through internal work. But the purpose is always personal and not the same for all of us.

Healing magic

All theories and views on life offer different approaches and maps of who you are and what you can do to develop yourself. But that's just what they are: only maps, although very useful. It is you, your experience, awareness and your presence within your own body which is important. The body and mind is a living system where everything is connected. However, sometimes it is difficult to keep in mind the logic and understand the cause and effect. Therefore, it is important to learn how to listen inwards and how to exercise awareness to understand different signs and symptoms. To have a higher perspective while the parts fall into place. In order to achieve this, well-designed exercises can be well-suited. It is in the mysterious connection between body and soul, matter and spirit, in the point where breathing, body and consciousness meet that healing magic can happen. This is also where you can perceive your potential and what is important for you and how you can serve your higher purpose.

> *The body and mind is a living system where everything is connected.*

Who am I? Where am I? Where do I come from? Where am I going? These are questions which mankind has been asking since ancient times. Today, more and more people are asking themselves what they can, and want, to give and do to contribute. How can I create harmony in my life and how will I become part of the solution for our planet?

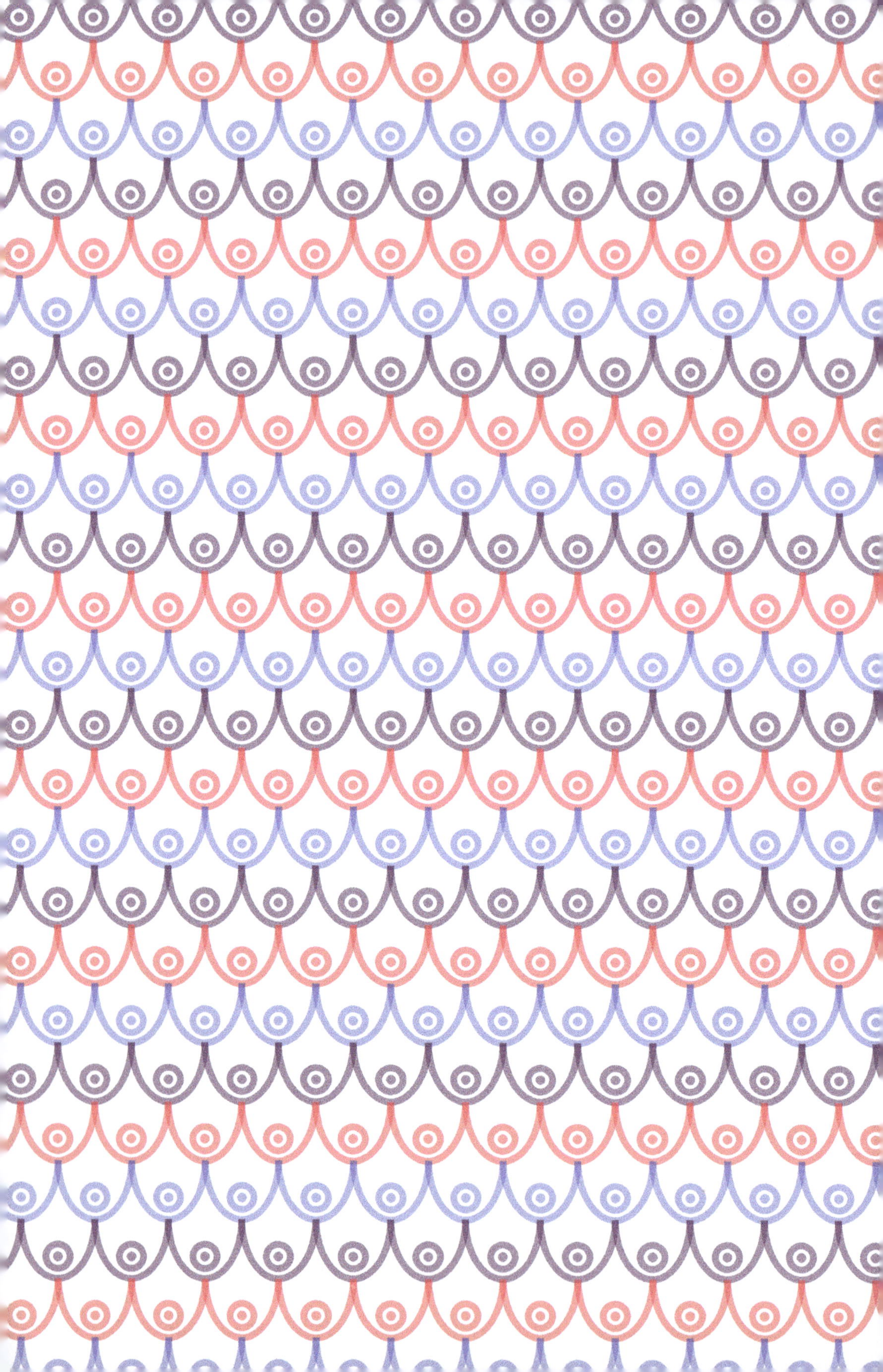

THE
FEMALE MYSTERY

Slow research on female anatomy

Various studies on feminine sexuality during the 1900's horrified some and surprised others. Meanwhile, they have helped many women. Even in modern times, the female orgasm, and ejaculation in particular, is often met with skepticism. In some circles, discussion about the "fountain orgasm" has been called the "UFO debate". Still in the early 2000's the female anatomy was not correctly described in anatomy books. It is reminiscent of the story when Columbus "discovered" America and called the indigenous population "Indians" because he believed that he had landed in India.

Since a woman does not need an orgasm or ejaculation in order to procreate, the interest in researching the topic has been weak and unprofitable. And since no one gets sick or suffers from not knowing about their erogenous zones or their inability to be able to get pleasure from them it has not been seen as a problem. Difficulties of measuring women's sexual responses have also offset interest, since they are largely an invisible, inner phenomenon. Ethical barriers have also existed.

Until recently the perception was that the woman's flow and orgasm had no function. It has however been shown that uterine contractions during orgasm with mucus from the cervix, causes the sperm to travel considerably faster up to the fallopian tube for fertilization. So even if an orgasm is not a must to achieve pregnancy, several studies have shown that the female orgasm includes some components that facilitate pregnancy. Older cultures, by contrast, have long known about the positive effects. More on this later.

Only in recent decades have discoveries been made about the actual size of the clitoris and about the female prostate. That women can ejaculate is now more or less accepted as a fact and the content of female ejaculate has been analyzed.

So what do these inquiries about a woman's anatomy, orgasm and ejaculation show? Tao sees it as important to understand how the body works to understand ourselves. Take the time to look more closely at the female body in an anatomical atlas. It strengthens the power of the exercises to have a clear picture of the various body parts and their functions.

Female anatomy

The woman's sexual organs consist of the vulva, vagina, uterus, ovaries, fallopian tubes, clitoris, urethra, prostate, glands, erectile tissue, pelvic floor muscles, blood vessels, nerves and erogenous zones. Overall, the female genitalia have proven to be larger and more complex than previously known, and may be measured by the scope and size of the male genitalia. Australian urologist, Helen O'Connell, was one of those who suspected that the anatomy books were not entirely complete. In the 1990's she had the opportunity to examine the internal parts of the clitoris in different women during autopsy. She found that it was much larger than previously thought, and in 1998 she published her findings in the science and technology publication The New Scientist.

There is great variation in the size and appearance of genitalia among women. This is documented knowledge in Tao and Quodoushka, where differences in anatomy are an entire theory regarding different body types and various ways of responding and arousal. For example, women have different depths and narrowness. The clitoris can sit at different distances from the vaginal opening and the G-zone can be located at various

Genital anatomy

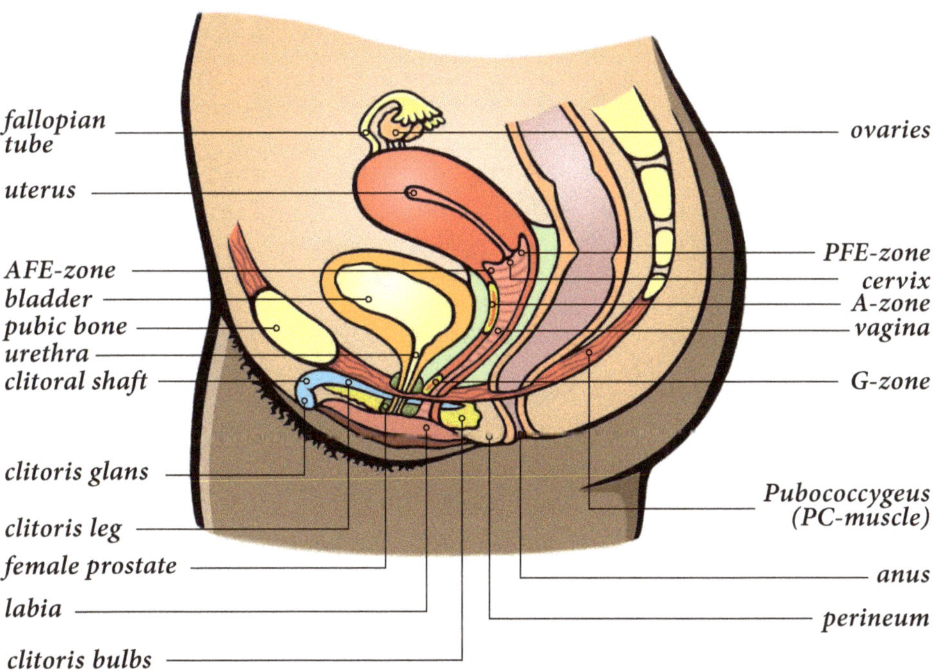

depths. These diverse manifestations are also linked to variations in the psyche and type of stimulation that works best. We are all unique in our expression, and yet still we are all the same.

Vulva

In medical terms, the woman's external genitalia is known as the "vulva", which means "cover" or "casing". The vulva is divided into the pubic bone, outer and inner labia, clitoral glans and perineum. The outer and inner labia vary in size and color and appear differently in different women. The inner labia form a cover over the clitoris, like a female version of a foreskin, called the frenulum. In the fold between the outer and inner labia are Fordyce glands that produce sebum so that the skin between the labia is constantly lubricated. The sebum has a whitish color and cream-like consistency. Production tends to be abundant in puberty and it then decreases in the adult female.

Vagina

The vagina is an approximately four inches long channel that connects the uterus to the external genitals and the outside world. Just as with male genitals, size varies, as we have already mentioned. The vagina channel is connected to the cervix and uterus, but also very intimate with the urethra and prostate, and close to bladder and rectum. The lower part is supported by the deep transverse perineal muscle, and above it is the levator ani muscle. The vagina has great elasticity and can be wider and longer during arousal and childbirth. It also includes several erogenous zones and has abundant blood vessels.

Similar to the oral cavity, the vagina always needs to be moist and lubricating fluid is secreted from the vaginal walls. Vaginal wall moisture comes from blood vessel liquid that penetrates the walls and forms specific lactic acid bacteria. This ensures the best environment with a pH value of 4.5 or lower, which means that undesirable bacteria and fungus cannot thrive in the vagina.

Secretion also comes from glands in the cervix as well as from the prostate gland around the urethra and the Bartholin's glands by the vaginal opening. Gland secretion increases during physical stimulation and arousal.

Urethra

The urethra is placed behind the pubic bone. It runs between the urethral opening and the bladder and is approximately one and a half inch long. The urethra empties between the clitoris and the vaginal opening. The passage of urine is controlled by the urethral sphincter and the pelvic floor muscles. Surrounding the urethra is the female prostate, an organ with glands and ducts that empties itself through the urethra when a woman ejaculates. Placed on the sides of the urethral opening are the paraurethral glands like a small triangular mucosa.

Perineum

The perineum is the area between the place where the outer labia meet, below the vaginal opening, and the anus. In the muscles and tissue inside the skin at the perineum there's a lot of nerves and blood vessels. So this area is often sensitive to touch and therefore an erogenous zone for many women.

Anus

Anus can be an erogenous zone for some women. There are also a lot of nerve endings in this area. Approach with care, never without concent, and safe hygiene.

Pelvic floor muscles

The pelvic floor muscles are composed of urogenital diaphragm, pelvic diaphragm and sphincters of anus, vagina and urethra. In Taoism, these strong pelvic muscles are sometimes referred to as the Qi muscle, or the orgasm muscles. You can read more about these muscles in a separate chapter later in the book (p. 129).

Pelvic diaphragm from above

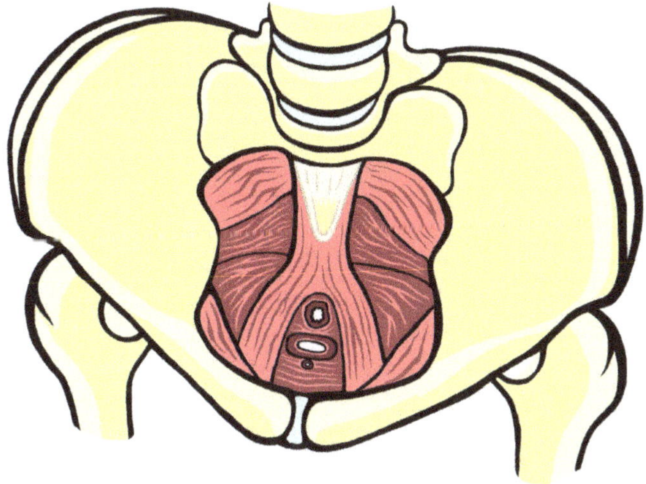

Uterus and cervix

The uterus is a hollow, pear-shaped muscular organ located in the female pelvis above the bladder and between the bladder and the rectum. It is within the uterus that the fetus develops during gestation. The cervix is the opening from the uterus into the vagina. The area around the cervix is called the anterior (front) fornix and the posterior (rear) fornix. The cervix contains mucus-producing glands that help to keep the vagina moist, clean and healthy. The secretions produce change of form and function with the monthly cycle. Each month the uterine lining is prepared to receive a fertilized egg. If no egg appears, parts of the blood filled lining are expelled approximately two weeks later. This is what we call menstruation.

The cervix itself can also be an erogenous zone. The approach need to be careful because the cervix doesn't like hard bumps, but softness, presence and stillness. Orgasms originated from here can create a fountain of bliss that bubbles up through your body. It will make you surrender to the divine. The orgasmic cervical nectar is white and thick and sometimes called "the liquid pearl". Tao says it is your deepest "inner heart". Some tantric's call it "the garden of love".

The uterus is often called "the womb space", and is seen as the origin of female power, filled with beauty, creativity and wisdom. It can birth much more than only physical children. In your womb you can plant seeds for your dreams.

Fallopian tubes

The fallopian tubes are two arcs that are connected to the upper part of the uterus. At the ends are funnel-like "hands" that capture eggs from the ovaries in a sweeping motion. Each month the ovaries release mature eggs, which float freely in the abdominal cavity before they are captured by the fallopian tubes. To allow fertilization to take place, the tubes transport sperm to the egg(s) and conception takes place within the fallopian tube. The fertilized egg is then carried to the uterus, which takes about three to four days.

Ovaries

Below the fallopian tubes are the ovaries, one on each side of the uterus. They are connected to the uterus through connective tissue. Women are born with millions of potential eggs in their ovaries, and in young women, there are about 400,000 eggs. Only about 400 of all of these will become finished eggs. During the fertile years one or more eggs are released each month from the ovaries. Perhaps you will only use one or two depending on how many children you have. The ovarian function is to provide us with these "egg mother cells" (oocytes) and also to produce sex hormones (progesterone, estrogen, and testosterone). Before cells become eggs they are called follicles and are embedded into the outer region of the ovaries, the cortex. The inner part is called the medulla. During ovulation, the eggs begin the journey to the uterus through the fallopian tubes where fertilization takes place. Without fertilization menstruation begins. This cycle takes about 28 days and is conducted in close cooperation with the pituitary gland and its hormones LH (Luteinizing Hormone) that triggers ovulation and FSH (Follicle Stimulating Hormone), which initiates the process.

Since every egg actually carries the potential of creating new life, we can understand that they are really holding an abundance of creative life force energy.

The female prostate

The female prostate gland is an organ around and along the urethral canal. It is about 1-2 inches and contains approximately 30-40 glands and ducts that are embedded in smooth muscle and erectile tissues (urethral sponge). The shape and location varies, but the meaty type with the widest part close to the urethral opening is most common. It has similar structure as the male prostate. It is also known as the Skene's glands and ducts.

The prostate functions is to produce and emit female ejaculate and PSA (prostate-specific antigen, an enzyme). PSA helps with dissolving the gel that surrounds the sperm before they can move freely. It secreate small amonts of ejaculate and large amount when sexually stimulated. One of the male prostate features is to continuously emit a very small amount of secretion, which is considered part of the urethra and prostate immune defense against infections. Most likely the same goes with the female prostate.

Another function is to produce hormones. The presence of serotonin has been confirmed and it is also thought to produce the female hormone estrogen and the hormone DHEA. Still, the gland is most studied in conjunction with ejaculation and not with other possible functions.

The Slovakian researcher, Dr. Milan Zaviacic (1940-2010), discovered that the female prostate has different shapes. In most women, it is a little wider towards the urethral orifice. The location, size and shape does not affect the sensitivity. Zaviacic did great work during two decades and his research is summarized in his book: "The Human Female Prostate: From Vestigal Skene's Paraurethral Glands and Ducts to Womans Functional Prostate" (1999). Since 2001, the female prostate has been an approved concept that is supported by "The Federative International Committee on Anatomical Terminology".

The prostate body can be touched from inside the vagina. You can actually both see it and touch it. If you look at the meaty area around your urethral opening, you see the beginning of it. Gush out with your pelvic floor muscles, and you will see even more. Then just follow from there with a finger inside. Often it feels like a distinct body, almost like hanging down from the front wall of the vagina, close to the vaginal opening. The great sensitivity on your front wall of the vagina, the erotic place we call the G-zone, actually comes from the prostate and its nerves. It is truly an erotic body and many today equate the prostate with the G-zone.

Bartholin's glands

Bartholin's glands are two glands located on the inside of the outer labia, slightly posterior towards the perineum. Two small channels from the glands open up on either side of the vaginal opening, and provide extra secretions in conjunction with sexual stimulation. Arousal and vaginal stimulation lubricate the vaginal walls with this clear secretion that has both a moisturizing and nourishing function. The liquid can be compared to the man's pre-ejaculate. The glands are named after Caspar Bartholin (1655-1738), the Danish medical student who "discovered" them.

Breasts and nipples

Breasts are central to a woman's experience of ecstasy and they can be the safest way to a woman's love, interest and devotion. They are your plus pole and are directly connected to both the heart and the genitals. A physical, loving touch without demands causes the oxytocin and a sense of togetherness to flow. In practice, this means that from the beginning the breasts are more important than your genitals. Through stimulation, hormones are secreted that open up the vagina and increase your receptivity. When a loving emphasis is placed on your breasts before penetration, it facilitates arousal.

Clitoris

The clitoris consists of a glans, with twice as many sensory nerves than the male glans penis. The glans is the part of the clitoris that is visible. On the inside there is a shaft and an inner portion extending up to four inches. The clitoris bulbs are lying horizontally and above the labia running on each side of the vagina and vaginal opening. A little further out towards the sides is the clitoris legs. The clitoral body consists of erectile tissue that swells during arousal. The body can be excited by stimulating the labia. You can massage clitoris legs and bulbs by massaging the muscles at the bottom of your pelvic floor, ischiocavernosus and bulbospongiosus (see p. 128). The clitoris body can thus be stimulated through pelvic floor exercises.

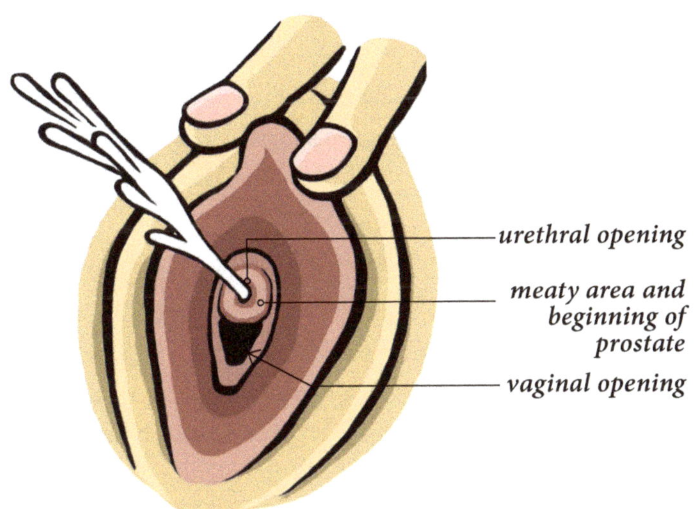

Stimulating the clitoris glans is the most common way to orgasm for women. The glans is not for nothing called the "bliss pearl". But I really recommend stimulation of the entire clitoris body to expand your experience.

Also the size of the clitoris can vary a lot. A survey of 200 women shows that the clitoris outer length varies by more than 25%. In autopsies, researchers have found that the internal parts of the clitoris can differ up to 100%.

G-zone

The G-zone is an erogenous area, as we have seen before, that is connected to the female prostate. It feels like a slightly ribbed area, about 1-2 inches inside the vagina on the front wall. This is where most of women feel it. In some women the G-zone is situated pretty far up and is out of reach for the fingers, in others can be experienced just inside the vaginal opening. But the whole body of the prostate can indeed be awaken to sexual pleasure.

This famous spot was named after Ernst Gräfenberg, a German gynecologist who "discovered" it in 1944. He called it the "erotic zone". It was Beverly Whipple, an American sex educator, that named it "the G-spot" after him. B. Whipple, A. Ladas and J. Perry made the G-spot known to the public through the book "The G-Spot and Other Recent Discoveries About Human Sexuality". It came out in 1982 and was translated into 19 different languages and has sold millions of copies.

Some now wants to call it the "goddess zone", while Taoists have long referred to it as the "black pearl of eroticism". Stimulation can lead to both strong pleasure and ejaculation. You can find it if you curl your middle finger into the vagina. Follow the prostate body, feel it and massage it gently. In the back of the prostate you may feel the texture ridged. You can try to do a "come hither" motion with your finger, while stroking the front wall of the vagina. Don't push hard and fast, start slow and conscious. It can take some time to wake up the sensitivity. It is easier to feel the pleasure zone when aroused. It can also vary from day to day. Sometimes this area can hurt or be numb. So take your time to explore, listen and feel into it.

The area that we call the "G-zone" was "found" in 1995 by Docent Olle Johansson of the Karolinska Institute in Stockholm. It happened by accident during research on the effect of microwaves on mucous membranes. A woman experienced symptoms in the vagina, which gave him reason to examine the lining of the vagina. He then saw this accumulation of nerves, that we now know belongs to the prostate, and to his surprise, even the nerve endings that probably contributes to the A-zone's sensitivity.

A-zone

The A-zone is a sensitive area in the vagina closer to the cervix. The actual anterior fornix is located next to the cervix and the A-zone is a little further down and towards the front wall of the vagina. Chua Chee Ann from Malaysia, educated in the U.S. and specialized in sexual health, described the A-zone in 1989. Touch stimulates rapid secretion of liquid in the vagina. Chee Ann also claimed that the liquid came from the prostate.

PFE-zone and AFE-zone

The PFE-zone (posterior fornix erogenous zone) is located below and behind the cervix, the vagina's deepest spot. The area is called the rectouterine pouch and also the Pouch of Douglas or the cul-de-sac, and is sometimes referred to as the epicenter or the "deep place". Stimulation may result in an intense orgasm. The zone can also be stimulated through the anus. The AFE-zone (anterior fornix erogenous zone) is located in front of the cervix and is often associated with the A-zone.

CUV complex

From the search for the G-spot came a new concept, clitourethrovaginal (CUV) compex. It is the relationships and the dynamic interactions between clitoris, urethra (prostate) and anterior vaginal wall during sexual stimulation and orgasmic responses. The whole area seems to be involved in our erotic adventures. These erotic bodyparts for sure share orgasmic nerves and blood supply in this erectile network of tissues.

P-zone

The area between the anus and the genitalia is called the P-zone (perineum). In Taoism it is the Hui Yin (meeting of yin). This area also has sensitive connective tissue that swells during erotic pleasure.

Nerves

Specific nerves are connected to different parts of the female genitalia. Each nerve is the co-creator of various unique orgasmic qualities and experiences and transfers information to and from the vagina through the spinal cord or nerve connections. That's why orgasms feel different. Below you can find the main erectile nerves described.

Pudendal nerve

This nerve is activated when the clitoral glans is stimulated. It also links to the clitoral body and the anterior third of the pelvic floor muscles.

Pelvic nerve

This nerve is activated when the vagina, prostate, urethra, cervix, uterus and rectum are stimulated and links to the rear two-thirds of the pelvic floor muscles.

Hypogastric nerve

This nerve transmits sensitive information and activity from the cervix and uterus. The nerve has links to the deepest part of the vagina and is probably important for vaginal lubrication and female ejaculation.

Vagus nerve

This significant nerve is especially associated with the vagina, cervix and uterus and is physically stimulated by penetration. The vagus nerve (the 10th cranial nerve), runs from the brain stem and branches out inside the rib cage and abdomen, and has connections to many of our inner organs, including the bladder, prostate and sexual organs. Cranial nerves are not found in the spinal cord, but go directly to the brain and brain stem from different parts of the body. This is the reason why a person with severed spinal cord still would be able to have an orgasm.

Tao and Tantra have long held the opinion that the vagus nerve is activated by relaxation and meditation and that it is important for both the mind and the senses. It constitutes a large part of the parasympathetic nervous system and is therefore essential for recovery. It also affects the throat and palate.

Hypoglossal nerve

The pudendal and pelvic nerves converge further up with a nerve called the hypoglossal nerve (the 12th cranial nerve), which controls the tongue. Heavy kissing can as we know be a real turn on.

These are examples of how different parts of the body are interrelated and interconnected via nerve pathways, and how they affect each other. The different nerves give different kinds of experiences when it comes to orgasms. Women can be wired differently. Some women's nerves branch out more in the vagina, others more in the clitoris, or cervix or perineum. If a nerve is compressed, for example by tense muscles, you can suffer from numbness. Even unawareness or poor contact with the genitals can affect the nerve response. A good investment to keep your sexual well-being up is to regulary do pelvic floor practice.

Brain

How the male brain reacts during orgasm was investigated in 1951 (admittedly with the technology available at that time). More than 50 years later, similar studies were conducted in 2004 when Dr. Barry Komisaruk, a neuroscientist from New Jersey, charted what it is that goes on in a woman's brain during orgasm. He was the first to use an MRI scanner and found activity at 30 different places in the brain, and also coupled the vagus nerve with perceived sensations in the genitalia. The study revealed that the differences between men and women were not that great. In both, the part of the brain that is responsible for logic and control is blocked. The emotional center is active, while activity in the anxiety center decreases. The number of hormones that exude strong feelings of love increase. The brain sends out orders to the genital muscles to contract. Wellness hormones and pain relieving hormones are secreted during orgasm. However, there are some differences between men and women. The woman's brain has a strong link to the part that is associated with pain and she can experience strong pain relief during orgasm. This probably also comes in handy when she is giving birth.

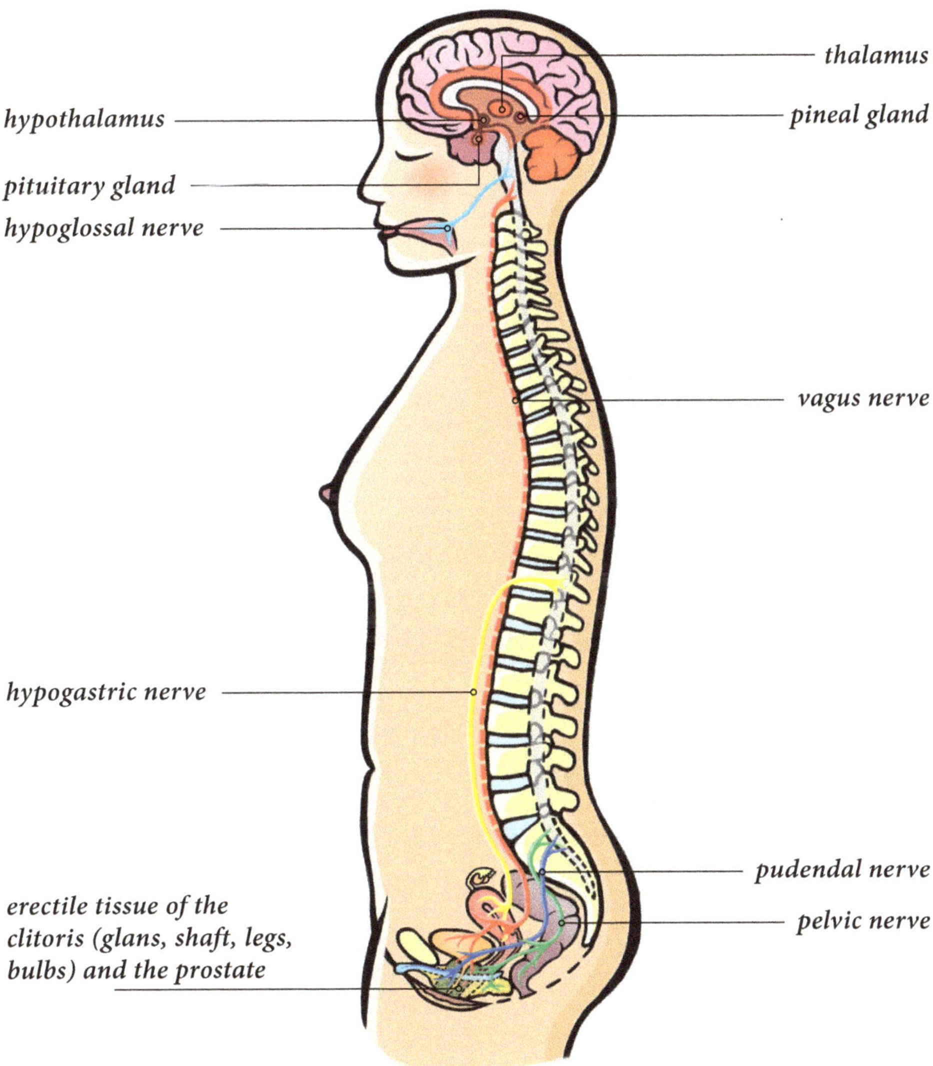

The brain, nerves and genitals are interrelated and influence each other.

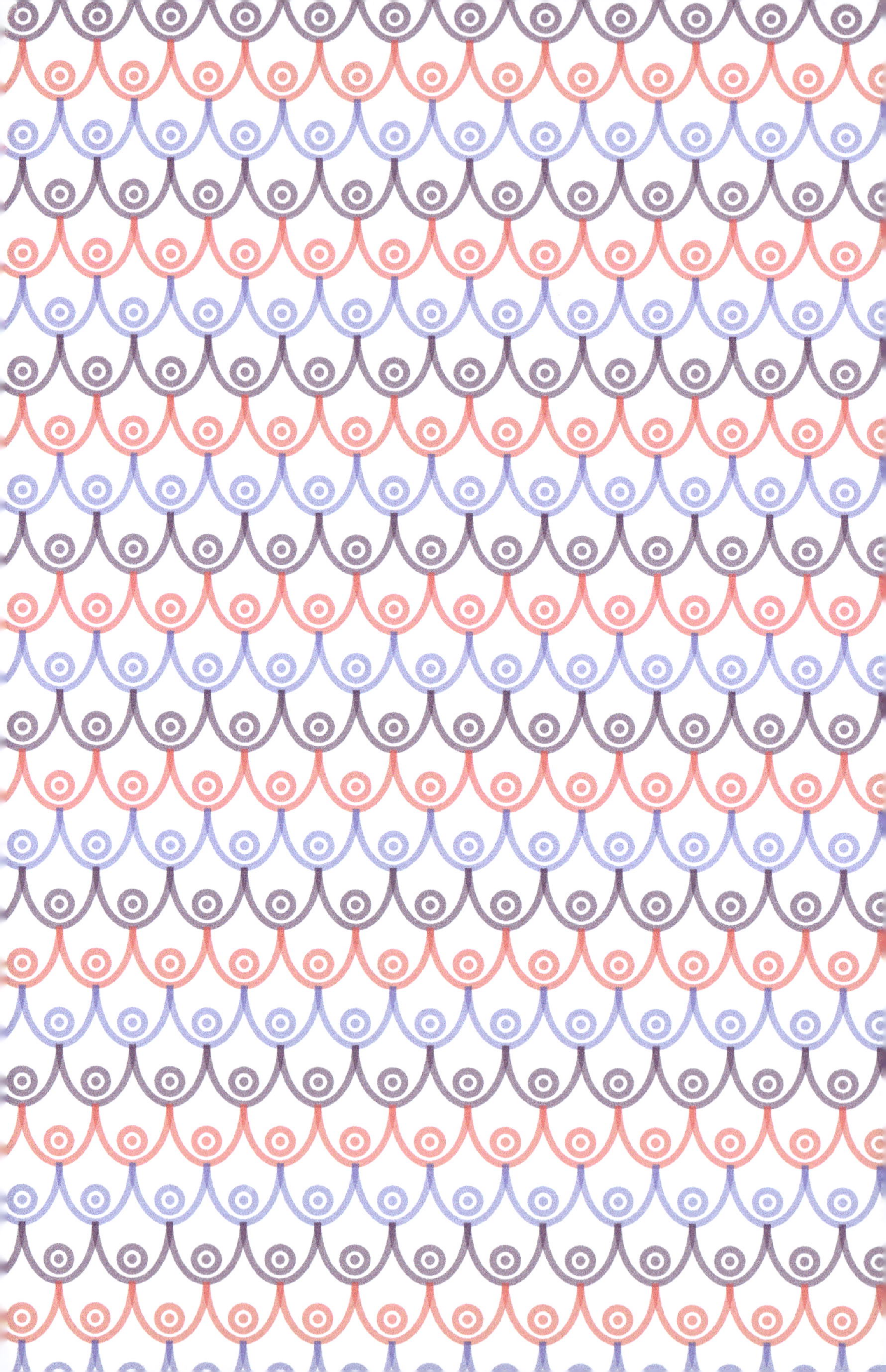

THE FEMININE ESSENCE

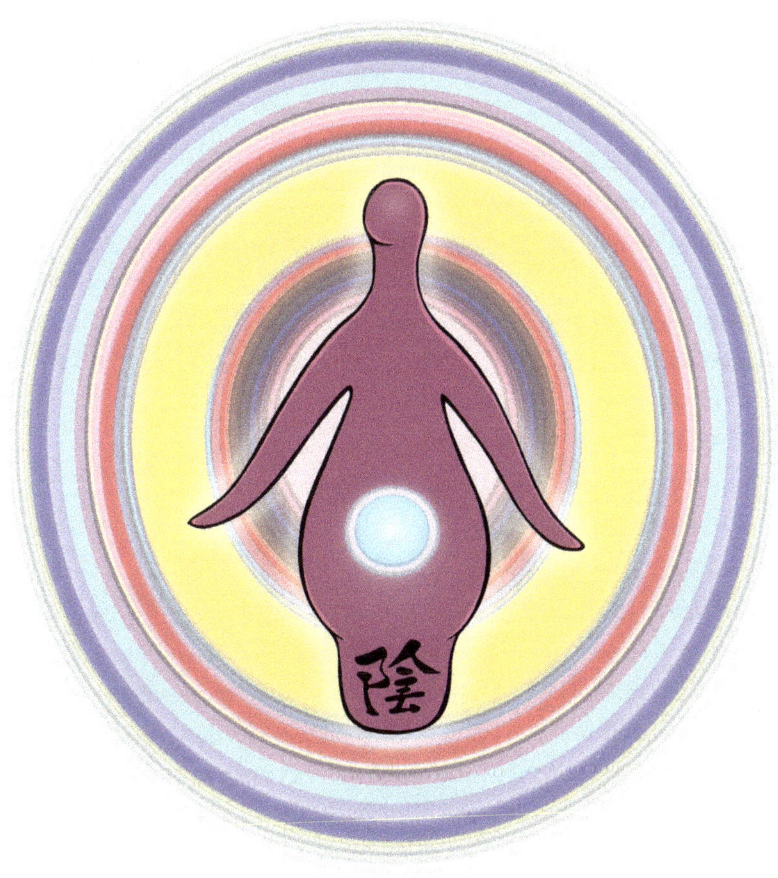

The female yin nature

As a woman, you are born in a woman's body and have a female perspective and consciousness. While this awareness includes both yin and yang, most women will approach life based on yin principles. This body and awareness is an expression of your feminine potential. Potential comes from the word potent and means "your capacity, your inherent power and your inner abilities". You may be aware of them or you may not, and maybe you've never thought about exploring them. A woman in balance with her nature has unlimited access to her feminine essence. Essence means that which makes someone or something what she or it is, an extract containing the essentials of this being.

Yin (the feminine) is symbolized in Taoist philosophy as an ocean or water and a woman is a living example of this. Water is constantly flowing, otherwise it becomes musty, it touches with tenderness and it, in its formlessness, fills up every space and is naturally drawn to the deepest place. Water takes on different expressions such as ice or steam, depending on its environment. Water can extinguish the fire (yang), and the fire could melt the ice or get the water to boil and evaporate.

> *A woman in balance with her nature has unlimited access to her feminine essence.*

To further deepen our understanding, we need to explore our yin nature and the aspects of ourselves such as deep, flowing, mysterious, earthy, darkness, body, silence, receptive, sensitive, adaptable, soft, fruitful, nature, indeterminate, instinctive, tireless and more. It is valuable to receive and begin to appreciate these qualities and to get in touch with what the feminine qualities stand for. It is not something you need to look for, but something that's already there. The feminine talks to us through feelings and our bodies. All you have to do is open up to this endless source of power. It can be easy to feel the essence of yin in silence and stillness, especially with other women around, but more difficult to describe it in words. Through the practices in this book you can explore your yin nature.

You are unique

All of these values are unique and it's about discovering what they mean to you. Our imprinting of religious dogmas and stereotypical gender roles and body ideals (not the least in the media) and our personal history have often not favored a free approach to our bodies and our yin nature, or our sexuality. In today's western society, women are independent and often provide for themselves. It is then easy to develop a surplus of yang energy, which is required for direction and action. In order to balance this surplus, we need to go inward and pay full attention to ourselves and build our true sense and connection from within. This is where you will find your essence, not by searching for it on the outside. Based on this inner connection, we can meet the world while retaining our yin nature. Strengthening yin is not about "freeing" yourself from men (yang) but rather about being closer to and nurturing your feminine essence. Freedom does not mean that you become a copy of the male, but that you become yourself. When yin is allowed to blossom it becomes easy and natural to accept, absorb and to develop yang. It is in this knowledge and respect for differences and polarity where both attraction and balance arise. An approach that goes hand in hand with your own self-acceptance and inner balance between yin and yang. We are in need of both, but as a woman you can find many keys to this through exploring and integrating your yin nature in depth.

> *When yin is allowed to blossom it becomes easy and natural to accept, absorb and develop yang.*

Everything in nature contains duality and works out of yin and yang (receptivity and activity, giving and receiving, support and challenge etc.). It is like two opposites in a unit which creates a force field, forces that can not exist or experience anything without each other. It is the same for the female and the male. Yin and Yang need, complement and balance each other. Being only receptive leads to passivity. Only being active becomes a meaningless action. When in contact with both yin and yang, you become receptive to your inherent creative power and ready to fertilize and take action. You will be responsive to your yang sides without losing the connection to your feminine power. A genius is one who can hold opposites. How does yin and yang interact within yourself? How does this reflect in your relationships?

Power games

Sometimes we play different power games to win each other's favor. A woman who has not gotten power from her inner and her yin nature may play on emotions and create dramas in her relationships with men. Inside, she feels insufficient and uncertain. She can use her sexual cunning to manipulate the man, while preventing herself from expressing herself naturally. Perhaps she chooses to have sex because of her longing for a partner or physical needs, and not because she really wants to. This behavior often leads to a sense of emptiness and disappointment, feelings of anger and of being used. Attempting to satisfy unconscious needs leads to unrealistic expectations and can be unsatisfactory on all levels. This leads to her being pushed into a need to free herself and to separate from the man to feel better. This in turn leads to confusion and a desire to take fight. The separation gives a false sense of liberation and is a reason why many women feel drained of energy. By not listening to what's going on inside, she denies both her sexual and spiritual nature. You can't absorb and embrace yang as long as you compete with men and fight against the male aspects of yourself. War outside and war within. The other way around applies to men. Our relationships reflect us. Recurring themes in relationships often have their foundations in family constellations from our childhood or inherited patterns from generations back. You need to be honest with yourself and perceive what views you defend to create the inner conflict. We make feelings too personal. Part of the process is changing our focus and taking a more neutral standpoint. To absorb yang, the male, active and fertilizing, you need to be more receptive to your creativity, i.e. more yin. How can you become more relaxed and receptive in everything you do? How can that make you more balanced and creative in your relationships?

The example above is a generalization of many women today having a surplus of yang and often compare themselves to men and compete with other women instead of deepening their femininity and their sisterhood. There are of course many different ways of creating an imbalance between yin and yang. For example, some women drain themselves through a surplus of yin instead. Then you are probably too passive and too adaptable and have no direction at all in life. This is for you to explore.

Why not go out into life and experiment a little. Dare to throw yourself into the unknown and explore new ways of being. Try different yin qualities and see what different reflections and mirror images you receive back. What will be the difference if you are flirting with a man based on how you think you're supposed to act to be "right for him" (a focus on the exterior) or based on your feminine essence, based on yourself and based on what you like (a focus on your inner self)? Which is the most creative, playful and attractive?

Because the woman in many ways is also a mystery to herself, she needs to be seen and appreciated for who "she is", which many times solely involves a pair of alert ears and full attention and presence from someone. No suggested solutions are needed. The man in turn needs appreciation for what he is doing, and often wants solutions and goals to feel satisfied. The Taoist approach to our yin nature contains insights and wisdom that are well worth exploring.

Tao also counts body fluids to be part of our essence.

A beneficent elixir

The feminine essence is as well a beneficent elixir produced by the body. The erotic fluids produced by stimulation, arousal and ejaculation contains many useful ingredients. The substances that are excreted during orgasm are the body's own "medicine". They enable the parasympathetic nervous system to be activated which reduces the secretion of stress hormones and increases the proportion of well-being hormones. The blood pressure decreases, the heartbeat becomes slower and the breathing becomes deeper. It sure sounds like a sophisticated and well-functioning anti-stress cure, which you can take advantage of.

The Taoists have long known this potential of our feminine essence expressed through our orgasmic fluids. The Yellow Emperor's female adviser Su Nu called it "an essence composed of a woman's inner heart". The feminine juice is seen as an expression of her female essence and inherent naturalness. It is a result of hormonal balance, an awake and receptive genital area, and an acceptance of the fluids which are the natural expression of the female body.

The woman's erotic flows

Then how does this complex and ingenious system of physical functions and ecstatic fluids work? As we have seen in the anatomy, different types of flow occur when a woman gets excited. It is fluid from the vaginal walls and mucus from the cervix, Bartholin's glands in the labia produce secretions and the glands in the female prostate produce their secretions. A woman may also ejaculate and even "spray" or "squirt" out a considerable amount of liquid. Often the climax comes with the orgasm. Saliva, tears and possible secretion from the breasts are also counted among the female flows.

Common erogenous parts which stimulate these fluids are the clitoris, prostate, vagina, erotic zones, breasts, mouth, tongue, anus or other favourite body parts. It can of cource also be enough with an admiring glance or appreciative word from the right person, a loving gesture or the fragrance of excited pheromones.

There are reports of arousal and orgasm without genital stimulation. For example, women have described how they can achieve orgasm only through excitatory thoughts. Some call the mind our biggest erotic zone.

Orgasm

It's your birthright to feel pleasure and reclaim your ability to orgasm. You have the privilege of being born with the capability not only to procreate, but also to enjoy sex. Everyone does not achieve orgasm, but everybody, even though we can look a little different, have the physical conditions to succeed. Orgasm ability may be there natually from early age or is something you learn to conquer. In most cases, a woman needs to feel an emotional bond and connection to open sexually. First with herself and from there with a partner. Before this happens, it rarely pays off to stimulate her physically. For the man, the order is often reversed.

The experience of the orgasm is something amazing and almost indescribable. You are unique and have your own special experiences and knowledge. The ancient Greek meaning of the word orgasm is close to "swelling with moisture" and "being excited and eager". Sometimes it is described as an explosive pleasurable discharge or as an altered ecstatic state of consciousness. In some dictionaries, orgasm is only described as a number of contractions in the pelvic floor, in response to physical stimulation of the genitals. We don't know exactly what triggers the orgasm. The experience tends to go toward the more mysterious direction. For the mystery cults, love making was seen as a way of communicating with the divine or awakening and exploring the creational power.

What happens during arosal and orgasmic states?

During excitement, the clitoris and erectile tissues swells and blood flow to the genitals increases. The vagina is moistened and expands and the uterus rises. Different nerves are activated. Sensitivity increases and excitement spreads through the whole body. The body and hips wants to move. Breathing intensifies, the pulse heightens and salivation increases. During the orgasm, powerful muscle contractions start in the pelvic floor, both voluntary and involuntary. Potential ejaculation may occur. Inside the uterus, mucus is produced which comes out through the cervix and into the vagina. During ovulation the mucus is used to catch the sperm. The strong contractions in the pelvic floor

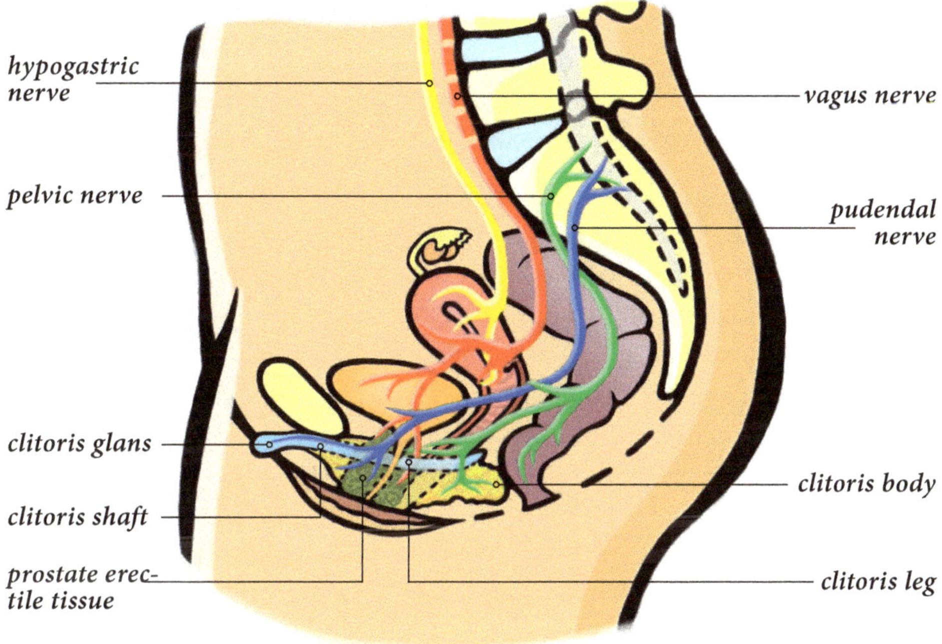

create an internal pressure in the uterus and the seed is caught in the suck-back. Different hormones are excreted before, during and after orgasm, including estrogen, testosterone, oxytocin, prolactin and DHEA. Even the pleasure experts dopamine and serotonin and the endorphins are active players. These are all substances that make you relaxed and filled with energy. Several areas in the brain that control emotions, behavior and muscles are activated. The pain threshold is raised and the immune system is activated. The proportion of beneficial negative ions increases. The body not only emits fluids but also transmits orgasmic energy, a significant psychic and spiritual power. The feeling and the experience are subjective and are part of the more mystical. They are beyond your control and beyond thoughts and words and time and space. With sexual Qigong you can stimulate and take charge of this orgasmic healthy and healing energy, both subtly excited energy and more aroused energy. The Tao practice help you prepere the body to recieve, transform and build the energy.

Different types of orgasms

Nowadays, we talk about several types of orgasms, such as clitoral orgasm, G-zone (prostate) orgasm, vaginal orgasm, mixed orgasm (clitoris and/or other zones), fountain orgasm (ejaculation), full body orgasm (orgasmic energy spread throughout the body), multiple orgasms (several in a row). There are also different levels depending on how energy rises in your body and affects your chakras (a term originating from yoga, meaning wheel or circle), different energy centers throughout our bodies. The orgasm can be anything from explosive and flowing to imploding and more subtle.

No matter what erogenous zone you are stimulating, in the Taoist practices you will learn how to lift the sexual energy and how to spread the orgasmic power up through your chakras and into your body. It expands your experience of enjoyment. The effect of moving the sexual energy upwards is unexplored here in the west but well-known in Tao and Tantra. Sexual energy is associated not only with pleasure and good health but also with a long life and the exploration of other worlds. It is rather strange that this most satisfying ability we have received has remained so uncharted. It is as if we expect the knowledge of our sexual potential to exist by itself. Unfortunately this is not always the case. But as with so much else, it is knowledge, understanding and practice that provide you with skill. A lot of sexual difficulties are not medical issues but a lack of information and sexual education.

Directing energy inwards and upwards in the body and along the spine helps it reach the pituitary gland and the pineal gland, the endocrine glands in our brains. They are sometimes called ”The Master glands” With these we guide and create our flows and our erotic and creative expressions. Through the ability to guide energy in combination with feeling safe, relaxation, deep breathing, awareness, bodily awareness, presence, will, intention, love, feelings, ability to surrender, opening your heart and investing in yourself, you will create different levels of intensity in your orgasm.

But, out of a purely genital physical functional perspective, we can divide this into these three major variants:

Clitoral orgasm: Stimulation via clitoris. No penetration needed. Rhythmic muscle contractions mostly in the frontal pelvic floor. The pudendal nerve becomes active through thousands of sensitive nerve endings in the clitoris.

G-zone orgasm: Stimulation of the prostate and the G-zone through the front wall of the vagina. Combines contractions in the pelvic floor and uterus. If with ejaculation, the vagina is pressed down as the muscles pump and push towards the vaginal opening. Sometimes it can even be difficult to keep something inside. The pelvic nerve as well as the vagus nerve is activated.

A-zone orgasm: Full penetration and stimulation of multiple zones, including the A-zone, AFE-PFE zones and cervix. All the muscles which facilitate orgasm are activated, strong contractions in the uterus and several orgasm nerves in the area are affected. The cervix opens and closes with a ”sucking” feeling when the uterus pulses.

Explore your erotic potential

Everybody can expand their ability to enjoy sex. The key to your pleasure awaits within you. The premise is just that you are interested and willing to find out how. The best way is to start exploring and investigating your erotic body parts. What is your relationship with your gender? What is your genital sense of self? What do you look like? Take a mirror and have a look at your genitals. Can you locate the entire clitoris and get a sense of your prostate and cervix? Find out what you like and what works for you. What is your body longing for? Let curiosity guide you and see, feel, touch, listen and try your way forward. Don't rush into arousal, slow down, use mindful touch and a self-loving attitude and approach. Part of your healing and development is to fully accept your sexuality and your body's appearance.

In Deborah Sundahl's book ”Female Ejaculation and The G-spot” there are plenty of concrete and exciting tips for those who want to deepen their physical explorations, including learning how to ejaculate. The whole body of the female prostate can be awakened to its full potential. Your whole womb and vagina can relax and open up to you. There is so much healing and love inside this treasure. Your ”inner heart” is full of pleasure, feelings and wisdom.

Remember that if you've lost contact with your sex and inner pleasure parts you can feel numb or there can even be pain. Trauma or abuse can be reasons for avoidance as well as pain. You need to spend time with yourself to help the body reawaken it's feelings, sensations and sensitivity. Take your time. Give your inner heart attention, acceptence and appreciation. If you are met with overwhelming emotions, seek professional help. It has also been proven that just talking about sex with other women improves sex life. So don't wait around, start sharing with your friends or find a group that can empower you in sisterhood.

The practices further will help you to create a space inside where you can hold greater awareness and acceptence of your self. A space where you can hold your own process and include everything that you are, including unpleasant emotions, or feelings of shame and guilt around your sexuality. When you can be comfortable whith the uncomfortable transformation happens.

Female ejaculation, is it possible?

Yes, it is possible, even if far from all women ejaculate, nor is it necessary to do so to have a satisfying sex life. Some people do it naturally and others have learned how to. Most often, a woman ejaculates in correlation with the orgasm, but not always. The ejaculation doesn't necessarily need to make an orgasm stronger or more satisfying, but many experience a sense of relief in the pelvis. Some of you will start ejaculate just knowing it is permitted, possible and natural. Many are already ejaculating, but just don't know it.

We do not know why some women may get an ejaculation and others might not. Regardless of the explanation behind female ejaculation, it is most likely something that the vast majority can learn how to do. This is an anatomic ability we are born with. Many have no awareness of how female ejaculation happen or what it is. Everybody should know what they do, and that female ejaculate is not the same as vaginal lubrication or urine. Female ejaculation is a powerful, beautiful, mysterious and a natural sexual response of the female body.

Here is an attempt to summarize a few milestones in history, some of the western research and the Tao approach to female ejaculation.

It is not pee!

First we have to clarify this; it's not urine, and it's not coital incontinence. The feeling of needing to pee during arousal is usally the urge to ejaculate. Many women stop the ejaculation since they're unsure whether or not the fluid may be urine. Go to the toilet before making love to get rid of insecurity. Or they may have been shamed in their early years when they've ejaculated. Over time, this habit of stopping the flow makes the muscle lock up and the behavior becomes automated. Too tense or too weak pelvic floor muscles can prevent ejaculation. But all this has probably contributed to the doubt about female ejaculation and its existence.

Views on female ejaculation in early cultures

The knowledge of the female ejaculation is not new. Different cultures around the world have known about its existence and described it as natural, normal and sometimes both sacred and healing. As early as 2,500 years ago, Chinese scientists and philosophers called the female fluids sacred and essential to life. They called it the "three sacred waters", three types of emission. The first water comes with arosal and deepens and widens the river. The second increases excitement and the flow of the river. The third comes with the orgasm which causes the river to flood and give birth to life and nourishment.

2,000 years ago, in Kama Sutra, the Hindu art of love, the ejaculation was described as the female seed, which continues to flow throughout the sexual intercourse. The nectar of the gods, amrita, was honored as sacred 1,000 years ago within the Indian Tantra. It is also recommended to drink these secretions called "amaroli" since they contain several healthy ingredients such as hormones, vitamins and minerals.

As far back as 600 BC - 200 AD the Greeks and the Romans knew about female ejaculation. They called the inner labia, where the fluid comes from, "nymphaea, the water goddess". The erotic flows, both female and male, were called the "liqueur of life" and were believed to be renewing and essential for reproduction. In Greek mythology, the flows were called ambrosia, which means immortality and served as the food of the gods.

> *The female fluid was described as natural, normal and sometimes both sacred and healing.*

The term the three sacred waters can also be found on the American continent, in the shaman teachings of love, Quodoushka. Vaginal secretions and dewdrops of the uterus are mixed and then called the "mist of the red jaguar". When the dewdrops are mixed with the ejaculated fluid, it is called the "venus river", filled with the elixir of life. This is seen as a reflection of the female life force. The river contains healthy and life-enhancing hormones and minerals. Ejaculation also represents the woman's ability to use her masculine active and fertilizing side, as well as being able to be a free, individual and autonomous woman, owning her orgasmic power and potential.

Even on the African continent, in Rwanda, up until this day, they accept and talk about the "sacred water". They see the sacred waters of female ejaculation as a very important ingredient of a sexual relationship. In Micronesia and the south pacific they call it "spray the wall".

Western views on female ejaculation

Female ejaculation has been portrayed in various ways through time and experts and researchers has been critical. Despite many convincing studies not all agree. While many have continued to believe it to be a modern myth, several investigations showed the opposite, and many women have been telling us about their experiences.

In 1672 the Dutch Reinier De Graaf (Dutch anatomist, 1641-1673) spoke of the ejaculation as something that sprays out of the woman. He saw the female prostate as the source.

In the 1950s, Ernst Gräfenberg (1881-1957) reported that stimulation of an area on the front wall of the vagina leads to the release of some kind of transparent fluid from the urethra that is not urine.

In 1981 Addiego and Whipple did a case study to once and for all prove that female ejaculation does exist. They biochemically analysed the fluid and confirmed that it was not urine. It contained PSA and therefore it may come from the female prostate. Just as men have a prostate-specific antigen, women do too, and this is a marker for scientists to recognize female ejaculate. From here modern research took off. Since then, many studies and several books have been published on the subject.

In 1982, Beverly Whipple (Whipple, Ladas & Perry) made female ejaculation known to the greater public through the book "The G-Spot", mentioned earlier.

In 1983 Alice Ladas et al. (American sex therapist) interviewed 400 women and documented their stories on sexuality and ejaculation. They summarized the resesarch and made it available to the public, and highlighted the female ejaculation. They wanted to give women knowledge of their own bodies and reduce any feelings of guilt and shame.

The, in its time, controversial writing "Eve's Secret: A Revolutionary Perspective on Human Sexuality", written in 1987 by Josephine Lowndes Sevely, described both the true face of the clitoris, prostate and the ejaculation. Already 1978 she wrote an article on the subject (with Bennett).

Dr. Milan Zaviacic, from Slovakia, has in his two decades of studies (1980s and 1990s), acknowledged the recognition of the female prostate as a fully functioning female organ and he examined its structure and the ejaculate fluid down to its cellular level. He stated: *This prostatic tissue is a new erogenic zone for females. It participates in the female ejaculation phenomenon, in which the female prostate is stimulated indirectly.* He also indicated that a small amount of ejaculation seeps into the vagina. This is possible since the urethra and the prostate share a wall within the vagina. If glucose is absorbed into the vagina from the ejaculate, it can create a favorable environment for sperm on its way to the egg. In this way female ejaculate may facilitate fertility. Dr Zaviacic's studies also indicated that female ejaculate may provide a soothing protective agent for the urethra, and holding back the ejaculation leads us to losing this advantage.

Dr. Francisco Cabello, a sexologist from Spain, did a study in 1997 which sugggested the possibility that all women ejaculate but they are not aware of it. This was explained by the fact that these women ejaculate in smaller amounts or that the ejaculate dissapears retrograde up into the bladder instead of being ejected. The theory is that if a woman holds back the ejaculate it will retrograde, and come out with the urine. In his study he found higher PSA in the urine sample after orgasm even if they did not ejaculate. Some have even speculated that retrograde or holding back ejaculation may contribute to bladder or urinary tract infections in women.

What does the female ejaculation contain?

Several studies in recent decades have confirmed the content of the liquid. They have found that the amount of fluid varies, from a few milliliters to several centiliters, and even up to a liter. The ejaculation can occur several times during intercourse. There may be small amounts of fluid throughout the sexual excitement, or a heavy jet of fluid that is ejaculated from the urethra. The fluid is a clear and watery texture or can be milky and whitish.

Taste and smell can vary slightly with the menstrual cycle and from person to person. The flavor can be anything from salty to fresh and a little earthy, but often the liquid has no clear taste or smell at all. The ejaculation fluid from a woman contains no sperm cells but is other than that the same as the ejaculation of a man; PSA (prostate-specific antigen), glucose, phosphate, enzymes, hormones, minerals and trace amount of urine. It is more basic (higher than 7 pH) than other fluids that come from the female genitals.

Where does the fluid come from?

The main origins for the female ejaculation is the female prostate. The glands of the prostate, produce and emit the fluid which is released into the urethra. The fluid is usually clear and watery, but can be witish.

Then there is a second theory, which is that fluid originate from the kidneys. This may be associated with a process that triggers the hormone aldosterone to be secreted from the adrenal glands during sexual arousal. It creates a fluid that collects in the bladder and releases out via the prostate and urethra during the ejaculation. This type of emmission is linked to the greater amount of ejaculate, and to the term "squirting". At present, there is a lack of facts regarding this theory. Both type of fluids can be excecreted during the same occation.

Squirting versus ejaculating

According to Gary Schubach (2001), who wrote his doctoral thesis on female ejaculation, there are two known types of female ejaculation. One is a milky withish liquid and comes in small to moderate volumes. The other is a watery liquid, called squirting or gushing, which can occur in a variety of volumes from an unnoticeable dribble to a wetness large enough to soak the sheets. The fluid has no odor or visible color and do not has any visual resemblance to urine. It contain traces of PSA and a lower amount of urine markers. Schubach said: *My theory is that the composition, as well as the color and odor of the ejaculate, is being affected by extreme arousal and the release of the hormone aldosterone.*

Although the researchers were surprised by the PSA value, in the volumous watery ejaculate, some chose to describe the phenomenon of squirting as "deluted urine". This missinterpretation lead to United Kingdom's sexist ban on female ejaculation and squirting in pornography. The interpretation that it was pee made it obscene. This is a clear reflection of our culture's ignorance of female sexuality. It was easier to explain the phenomenon as a dysfunction than to open up to a greater understanding of woman's sexuality.

This was done despite the fact that many women expressed experiences that contradicted the researchers conclusions. Most women who experience ejaculation, more often have the clear and watery fluid, and they all confirm it is definitely not urine. This is also confirmed by Deborah Sundahl, who tought thousands women to ejaculate for over three decades. Try for yourself next time you ejaculate, look, smell and taste it.

But even if the scientists call the more profuse emission deluted urine, they admit that it's a product of sexual stimulation. Female ejaculation is a normal sexual response and the prostate is the main source, and there may be other origins. Whatever the science comes up with, it is obvious that, like crying tears, the genital glands seem to be able to create an abundance of erotic flows when women get loved and exited. No matter what any expert is saying or what any research is showing, let it never limit what is possible, nor define your sexual experiences. Remember that your experience is yours, there is nothing wrong with whatever you experience. So explore and share with other women and inspire each other. We just can't deny our own and thousands of women's sexual experiences.

A quote from Deborah Sundahl: *Choosing to ejaculate gives women freedom to use the anatomical ability she was born with in order to increase her sexual pleasure and health. Let it flow!*

The three sacred waters

How does Taoist sexology view the female ejaculation? It involves the term "the three sacred waters", a theory where these waters each have their qualitites and their gate that activates them. Awareness of them will help you activate the different expressions of their nature. The first water comes from stimulation of clitoris, the second from stimulation of the G-zone (prostate) and the third from stimulation of the A-zone and cervix.

1st gate: The first water is described to come during stimulation of clitoris, preferably the entire clitoris body, which also activates the female prostate glands. This sacred water essence is thin, may be whitish, and the taste can vary with the menstrual cycle. Deep breathing, nipple massage, relaxation and an open heart are keys to open the first gate. It prepares the body for deeper journeys.

2nd gate: The second water is stimulated through the G-zone, the grooved area slightly inside an on the front wall of the vagina, on the back of the prostate. This is the most common way for women to ejaculate. This sacred water essence is released from the kidneys through the bladder via the prostate and urethra. The liquid is thin and clear. Dedication, feeling safe, intimacy and emotions opens this second gate. To breathe deeply, opening the throat and making a sound deep inside the body can facilitate this water. Pelvic floor muscles may push out during orgasmic contractions. It clears the way to go even deeper. The whole body is shivering with pleasure.

3rd gate: The third water is linked to stimulation of the A-zone and the area around the cervix, which requires deeper penetration. The glands of the cervix is the origin of this sacred water. The result is a deep vaginal orgasm with thick, sticky and white-like secretion. Powerful sexual healing and spiritual connection can be experienced, or an intense opening of the heart and overwhelming feelings of love. The heart may bursts open with tears of joy. The key to the third gate is to allow yourself to fall into the mysterious endless ocean of pleasure. Penetration need to be slow, soft and loving. It opens the thrusting channel and connects you deep inside your core, like a fountain of exuberant bliss.

"Sexercise" can reduce the risk of heart attacks.

The first and second waters can be triggered without orgasm, but according to the Taoists, the energy can leak out as a result. The orgasm should be part of the practice of the three waters for best outcome. While, on the contrary, you don't need to ejaculate to take advantage of the benefits. In addition to the pleasure, the result and reward are an increased libido, released stress, better sleep, deeper relaxation, and an increased ability for sexual enjoyment, as well as a healing and sacred experience. Good conditions for vaginal lubrication and ejaculation are to have a flexible and relaxed pelvic floor muscle, to be multi-orgasmic and to have enough testosterone and an optimal amount of estrogen as well as an open mind that can connect with and touch your inside.

Perhaps this only sounds strange or unachievable and impossible to cope with. It's not supposed to discourage you, but rather inspire and tell you about different approaches, choices and opportunities. We can develop ourselves by becoming more erotically skillful. Sexual education and information promotes self-confidence. Strive to be open to all possibilities and more awake and alive in your body and vagina. This way you support the three sacred waters flow harmoniously and naturally. And don't believe anything. The knowledge must be tested before it becomes true wisdom. Try and see how and what works for you.

Sex for the sake of health

The fact that sex affects health is discussed openly today. Research has confirmed that orgasms increase our well-being, strengthens the immune system, reduces stress, improves sleep, and can relieve PMS. Studies show that many people masturbate to sleep better, reduce stress or to relieve pain. Orgasmic flows also have a balancing effect on the hormone system, including the secretion of the PEA love hormone (also found in chocolate), analgesic endorphins, the happiness hormone DHEA and the touch and feel-good hormone oxytocin, which in turn stimulates the pelvic floor and various other lust-filled sex hormones.

That love-making is healthy is sometimes given attention to in the media. An article in the Swedish newspaper Metro, spring 2010, could tell us that, according to the UK Health Agency NHS, "sexercise" can reduce the risk of heart attacks and prolong life, strengthen the immune system and also reduce the risk of various diseases. An article in the LA Times in Los Angeles tells us that orgasms strengthen health by releasing DHEA, which keeps the arteries clear and helps the heart. And a British study of 1,000 people has found that two orgasms a week reduce the death rate by half compared to those who eroticize less than once a month.

THE PATH OF LIFE

Natural cycles in life

Nature and life are constantly changing and undergoing different cycles. The seasons speak clearly about how life, death, transformation and regeneration interact. As women we go through different stages of the life cycle, from being children and teenagers to becoming fertile women. Then comes the menopause, when we move into being a full-grown woman, then lastly going on into old age and hopefully becoming the wise grandmother. Previously, civilizations had transitional rites for the various stages of development so that humans could more easily adapt and continue to develop. You can not change the life cycle, only approach it with respect and humility. You can choose to acquire knowledge and have a curious attitude and keep up with the changes.

Menstrual cycle

Throughout your long fertile span, you have the opportunity to conceive children every month. During ovulation, your estrogen levels are the highest and you usually feel the most attractive and willing. Approximately two weeks later, comes your period which, according to many, can be a time for cleansing and contemplation and an opportunity to look inwards. It can be a monthly possibility to heal and take care of unprocessed emotions. You remove emotional debris with your menstrual blood.

The moon's cycle and your menstrual cylce are in synchrocity. This is no coincidence and ancient cultures understood this. The body reflects cycles and movements in our environment. Traditionally, Tao links bleeding to the new moon (yin, downward force) and ovulation to the full moon (yang, upward force). But many women's cycle is reversed; they menstruate on the full moon and ovulate on the new moon. It is sometimes claimed that they use their sexual energy for spiritual growth instead of reproduction. It is common to swing between these two cycles. The moon affects the water on the planet, and the water in our body (blood and emotions), and is linked to female power. Take time to sneak on your contact with this mysterious connection. To reconnect with the moon's energies and different faces is healing and rewarding, also to keep balance after menopause.

Some women have different recurrent problems with PMS in connection with menstruation. These ailments can be caused by a variety of things, ranging from unbalanced emotions and stress to obesity and hormonal disorders due to the environment or food. Also be aware that hormonal birth control prevents ovulation and creates disharmony. Even personality, displaced emotions, attitude and heredity can play an important role. During the exercises, we strive to develop self-knowledge so that you can create a strong foundation for maintaining your balance.

Natural birth control

Over the centuries, the approach to sex has been characterized by its child-producing function. Women's right to work in order to support themselves and the emergence of contraception in the 1960s meant a lot for women's liberation. But nothing good comes without the bad and the pill has been questioned. Therefore, I would like to say a few words about preventive options besides condoms. Natural birth control involves respect for the body and having an awareness of the pills' bodily and ecological side effects. One method involves that you investigate (feel and look) every day and note what kind of discharges you have. During a normal menstrual cycle of about 28 days, ovulation occurs on day 14, calculated from the first day of the period. When ovulation is in progress, the discharge is clear and wiry, it's a bit like egg white, and afterwards it's thick and white. This also can be noticed in differences in temperature: the days before ovulation there is a decrease in body temperature and afterwards it rises again. After 2-3 months of analysis you should know your body. More detailed approaches can nowadays easily be found online and it is both helpful and recommended to find a coach in fertility awareness, in for example the Justisse method.

The cervix produces different secretions during different parts of the cycle. A type of secretion plugs the cervix and prevents sperm from getting up there, another sorts away bad sperm. During a short period of time, a welcoming secretion will help the sperm through the cervix and into the oviduct. It's basically only during this time that you have the chance to conceive. However, there are other more clever secretion fluids that can "lock up" for sperm which hides in cavities. It happens at times that sperm lingers after intercourse in the pockets at the sides of the cervix, where the sperm can survive for up to five days.

The few days after ovulation to the last day of the period is the safest time frame and the risk of becoming pregnant is at its lowest. In order for the natural method to be as safe as possible, you should not have penetrative sex during the five days before ovulation starts and the three days after. If you want to get pregnant on the other hand, this is when you have the greatest chance to conceive. Correctly used, this method can be a natural alternative. It works best if you have a fairly regular cycle or if you take the time to understand how to interpret your secretions, basal temperature and the position of the cervix.

Even in Taoism, natural preventive control can be found. Through specific exercises, a combination of ovarian breathing, breast massage, squeezing exercises and a strong intention, you can stop ovulation and therefore stop menstruating. Like creating a premature menopause. This requires knowledge of one's body, dedication and regularity.

When you stop doing the exercises regularly, the ovulation starts again and the period returns. The traditional name of this kind of training is "slaying the red dragon". This was part of the traditional training to accelerate women's spiritual development. Attention and flow are turned from outer manifestation to an inner focus. When I practiced the above-mentioned exercises daily, the amount of menstrual blood decreased radically within a couple of months.

I don't recommend trying this process without great confidence or a teacher that can guide you. Normally it is only natural and healthy to menstruate, which also is a great opportunity to go inside of yourself and reconnect to your true desire and clear away what's in the way.

Menopause

How did the menopause transition go from something natural to being a bodily defect which should be addressed and cured with pills? When the first hormone pill appeared in the 1940s, the menopause suddenly became a medical problem instead of a natural transition. An industry that has since flourished. Today we are hopefully heading back towards a more humane and natural approach. The body naturally limits fertility to a certain period. As important as paying attention to the first period is to celelbrate when a woman enters the phase of life that begins when the period ends, the menopause.

Menopause, just like puberty, is a transition from one phase in life to another. As we age, ovaries produce less and less estrogen and progesterone. It is a gradual process that occurs between 35 and 55 years of age. The body switches from reproduction to a new orientation in life. The word, climacteric, also means – important turning point. The menopause is a term for the last menstrual period. The duration of the transition period, as well as the symptoms, vary considerably between different individuals. Physical symptoms may, but need not, consist of hot flashes, dry mucous membranes, sleep disorders, weight gain and more. You can also feel more emotional and have mood swings. When the body changes it can make you more vulnerable and unworked experiences and emotions or traumas may remind themselves. The time has come to make a closing. We all need to take a break periodically to review our values and ask ourselves if we invest our energy in what is really important to us. How do you want to continue living the rest of your life? On page 139 there is a ceremony you can try for greater clarity.

Hormones decrease, but there is hope

During menopause, the production of progesterone decreases by approximately 75% but of estrogen only by about 35-50%. The availability of male sex hormones also decreases. However, some hormone production continues for many years, especially in the form of androgen, in the interior of the ovaries, their marrow. These androgens, including DHEA, can then be converted to female sex hormones in organs such as the liver, kidneys, pineal gland, brain, as well as in muscle and fatty tissue. This is one of the reasons why women who enter menopause often put on extra weight. The fat cells simply want to help produce estrogen. The female body thus has the ability to make adjustments to the hormone balance even after going through the menopause. There is a lot that speaks for that the exercises in this book are beneficial in stimulating these extra resources, for example ovarian breathing. Then you make sure to cultivate your libido regularly. The stone egg exercises help the vagina continue to produce secretions, even for women who have entered the menopause. There is nothing physiological that says that the desire for sex should decrease. However, brittle mucous make sex more fragile.

> *The female body thus has the ability to make adjustments to the hormone balance even after menopause.*

When you have sex or get an orgasm, hormones elevate your lust. Women who continue to be sexually active after the menopause keep their mucous membranes moist and limber longer. If you stop you may disconnect from your body and sexual energi, which actually is your life force. Many menopausal women experience a lack of sexual lust and might think it has disappeared. Then you have to rediscover it. It will be a choice you need to make. Most likely you will not just wake up one day and find your sexuality to be fully awake again. It takes what it takes, it's your choice and dedication. You may want to explore deeper needs for closeness and intimacy as well as new ways to have sex. Maybe your marriage is about to be dissolved or deepened. Masturbation can also be a good thing, or do things for the body that you really enjoy. Maybe you want to caress yourself and make self-pleasure and orgasm a discipline? Once a week or more? Caress yourself and try the self-pleasure exercise on p. 112.

The menopause is a physiological adaptation to a new phase, which in itself shouldn't cause any major unwanted symptoms. Perhaps it's our industrialized culture and lifestyle that is the biggest problem, coupled with a negative attitude. Attitude and approach is everything and really matters. Our biochemistry will affect the hormones. There is still much we don't understand about the hormonal change during menopause and there is therefore much left to explore. So be curious and explore where this process will take you. The womens body was designed to be a scorce of pleasure, joy, creativity, widom and well-being.

The golden eggs of wisdom

When the female flow after the last menstruation is no longer focused on creating children, it turns inwards, towards the heart. This is what the Taoists say; this is the time when you naturally begin to grow spiritually. From the production of eggs and blood, the Jing Qi, i.e. your sexual energy and your essence from the kidneys, is now turning towards the heart.

Many also experience a new greater sense of self-esteem, increased calm in the mind and greater peace in their hearts. Passionate sex becomes more focused on intimacy and closeness. According to Tao, the woman should also become more yang (outgoing, active and fertilizing) to balance the transition. Paradoxically, you get there by nurturing your yin (inward, receptive and creative) even more.

The shaman tradition describes how you, through the menopause, enter the full-grown woman's phase, becoming the wise woman who is dreaming for seven generations to come. The ovaries are now called "the golden eggs of wisdom". The flushes are seen as fast energy which want to be used and channeled. The focus is not to remove symptoms but to use the energy, changing your attitude, acquiring new intentions in life and creating a good design in alignment with the new visions. Be qurious, dedicated to your own process and co-create. That is a fruitful approach to this transformation which all women go through.

Before the menopause, it was the outer bark of the ovaries, that which produced eggs, that was the most productive. During menopause it is instead the ovarian marrow, their inner (even physically) that becomes more active. The ovaries do not "shrivel", which is sometimes claimed, instead they become the golden eggs of wisdom.

Our lifestyle creates an estrogen dominance

There are those who believe that it's not the lack of estrogen that is the biggest reason for PMS and imbalances during menopause, but the balance between progesterone and estrogen. Our lifestyle seems to contribute to an increase in estrogen. Two major advocates of this are Dr. Michael Lam, a physician and nutritional specialist from the United States who focuses on people who burn out as well as hormone balance, and Dr. John Lee, also from the United States, who has written several books on hormone balance and who was a popular lecturer on optimal health.

Much also points to exposure to several estrogen-like hormones through proteins in the meat we eat, through pesticides in vegetables and petrochemical compounds in plastic packaging, creams and soaps. Not to mention all birth control pills and synthetic estrogens and progesterones in hormone treatments which are flushed out into our water. Studies have confirmed changes in animals derived from estrogen in nature, including alligators where the females have very large ovaries and the males have very small penises. In addition to feminized animals, fish in Sweden have also been found to have high levels of synthetic progesterone. In Denmark, doctors wonder why puberty occurs increasingly early. In addition to all this, we are exposed to stress which exacerbates the adrenal glands, which leads to reduced progesterone production. Stress is probably one of the most overlooked causes of estrogen dominance. Obesity converts steroids into estrogen and other lifestyle problems such as an increased sugar intake, vitamin B deficiency and excessive consumption of coffee help to maintain the imbalance.

Protect yourself from stress

What is stress? Why are you stressed? And what happens if you expose your body to high levels of stress for a long time? In these times of constant threats of planetary disasters, pandemics, economic crises and general ignorance and unwillingness to take responsibility for what we know about ourselves and nature, it is difficult not to feel hopeless. In Sweden, we are culturally oriented to do good and we have a lot of 'musts' and pressure on us, both in family life and in work life. Also the uncertainty and feeling of not being able to influence affect our stress levels. The disconnection from the heart is instant, and fear and pressure is entering. We try in vain to control an uncontrollable world, or to avoid unpleasantries, which only drains the life energy and removes us from awareness even more.

> *Although the world is not always a peaceful place, it's possible to create harmony in your relationship to yourself and thus to your environment.*

The environment exposes us to stress through poisons, radiation and a lifestyle which may be forced upon us. All this creates a general state of physical, emotional, mental, spiritual and sexual tension. The pressure breaks down the life energy and does not allow it to circulate freely, either within ourselves or in interaction with our environment. During prolonged stress, the nervous system becomes less and less sensitive. Everyone knows that long-term stress is not good and that lack of recovery is devastating. Nevertheless, the first symptoms that start sneaking up on you, such as fatigue, insomnia and problems concentrating, are often overlooked.

The nervous system and the biochemistry under stress

Biochemically, we are well aware of what happens when the sympathetic nervous system is allowed to be active for a long time. The pituitary gland receives signals from the hypothalamus to mobilize all cells in the body to handle the "danger". The adrenal glands are ordered to produce stress hormones. Since many of the dangers we experience in society are constant and often unrealistic, the bodily system remains constantly ready to freeze, fight or flight, which eventually has devastating consequences. The stress affects the adrenal glands that are directly linked to your sexuality and your vitality. If the adrenal glands become completely exhausted, it can affect you very negatively and create major bodily imbalances, including lost sex desire. Should you burn yourself out it could in the worst case scenario lead to a total collapse. The digestion deteriorates and the ability of the immune system is lowered because all energy is used for defense in order to prevent the invasive threat. Stressed adrenal glands make you light sensitive, hypersensitive to sound, dizzy and decrepit. As the symptoms deteriorate, the risk of bodily inflammation also increases, as cortisol levels are affected. The kidneys are, according to TCM, the batteries of the body and it takes a long time to restore and repair them.

Rest and contemplation are literally vital. Everything is connected and is in constant motion.

Create time for recovery

Your attitude and ability to handle your thoughts and your environment are crucial to being able to respond to stress factors in a healthy way. Creating space for recovery is also fundamental. Because even though you can't directly affect the autonomic nervous system, you can do it indirectly by creating situations where your body gets a chance to recover. Then you can generate both awareness and energy, which you need to take responsibility and create action. My hope is that the knowledge and practices in this book will be an inspiration to you on your way to greater readiness for approaching life in a nurturing way. To find your way to create greater balance between yin and yang. Although the world is not always a peaceful place, there is the opportunity to create harmony in your relationship to yourself and thereby to your surroundings.

Finally

The Taoists thus describe your sexual energy, your orgasmic flows, and your female essence as an elixir of youth. They created exercises to cultivate life energy. Even if you don't have a partner or a relationship with an active sex life, it's still very valuable to be able to exercise your libido. Many spiritual teachings have perceived the sexual energy to be important and modern research also confirms that sexual activity is good for your health. Your glands and your hormone balance are also very important in this matter. Rest and contemplation are literally vital. Everything is connected and in constant motion. The exercises that follow can hopefully help you get to know yourself and your energy better. They show you how to develop your vitality, raise your awareness and ability to feel, awaken and guide your Qi and sexual energy and how to use it for your well-being. In addition, you will learn how to exercise your pelvic floor muscles, how to increase your sensitivity and your ability to have an even more enjoyable love life.

Physical practice is needed to move stuck energy and to support you to awaken to your inner essence. There is so much potential stored in the body. When you go into yourself, you also cultivate your energy body. Your soul connection deepens and you make space for the original spirit to take place in your heart again. Your highest potential is awaiting to be unfold. This is an ongoing process that happens in the present moment.

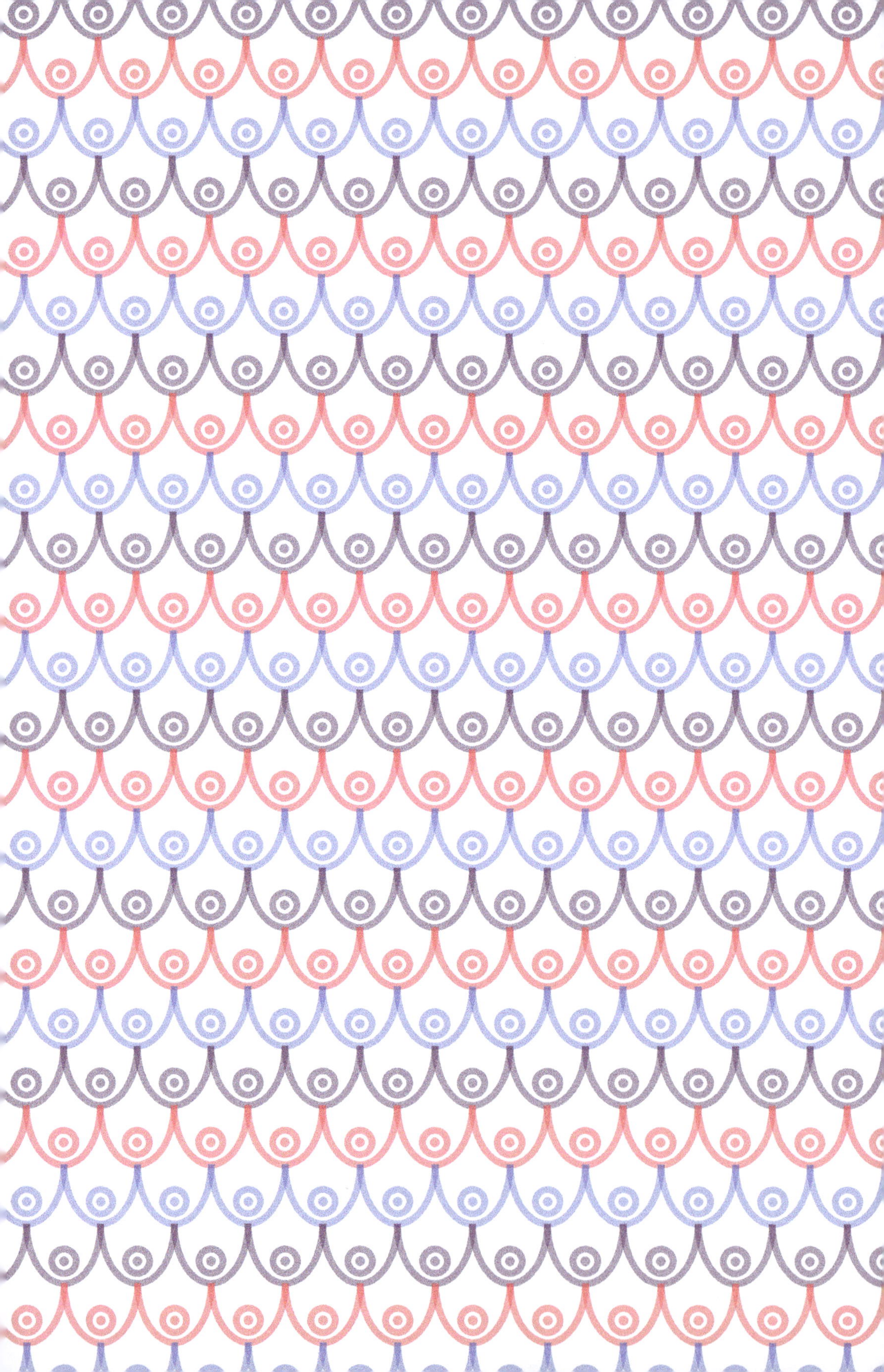

EXERCISES

Before the exercises

Several of the exercises that follow are internal guided meditations where you move your attention around the body with the power of thought. You use your awareness to guide the energy. With your mind you can lead Qi to any part of the body. It is beneficial that you keep an open mind and a curious attitude in your exploration. Keep in mind that when you focus inward you can use your breath to get in touch with different body parts. As a rule, you breathe in and out through your nose. Your inner eyes help you to see and your inner ears help you to listen to your inner world. You can rely on your presence and your intentions to make a difference. All exercises are designed to create or restore a natural flow.

Prior to each exercise I recommend preparatory exercises and sometimes also finishing exercises. The exercises build on each other to some extent, but all can be done individually. I do, however, always recommend starting with basic positions, exercise 1, to create a supportive posture. Finish with collecting the Qi you've generated, exercise 3, in order for the vital life force energy to be preserved.

Various reactions

In the beginning you may feel tired when you concentrate for a long time. But that feeling usually goes away and is a response to resistance or energy that comes into motion, as well as the habit of associating relaxation with sleep. You may also feel tingling, vibrating or prickly sensations when you release tension. Other reactions may be burps and yawning. If you get dizzy, then open your eyes and focus on your breathing and on your feet. Take your time and respect your limitations.

Emotional reaction

Sometimes memories with related emotions and history unravel. The recommendation is not to try to avoid the emotion or resist it, but to take on a neutral, observing and accepting attitude. Thoughts and feelings come and flow through you constantly, and they are part of your life energy, no matter what form they are taking on at the moment. Through these exercises and your presence, your unprocessed emotions can be transformed and restored to life-giving power.

NOTE!

If you are ill or not well, whether mental or physical, or feel unsure if an exercise is good for you, contact your doctor, other professional contact or speak with an experienced Qigong instructor.

EXERCISE 1:

Basic positions

Here's a guide to finding a good posture as a foundation, a good starting point and space within yourself, for both sitting and standing exercises. Your posture affects both your breathing and Qi flow. To have a special place or room where you do the exercises is also recommended.

Guide exercise 1:

Time: 5 min, sitting or standing

Purpose: Correct your posture ❤ Turn your attention inward ❤ Connection with heaven and earth

Standing basic position:

Stand with parallel feet, approximately hip width apart and with your toes straight ahead. Softly bend your ankles, knees and hips and relax your groins. Pull your tailbone in slightly between your legs so that the lower back is smooth and becomes straight. Let your arms hang down along the sides of your body and have an open feeling in your chest. Guide your sternum slightly forward and upward, to get your shoulders into place. Your chin is slightly pulled in to have your neck become an extension of the spine. Notice where the center of gravity is in your footpads and swing back and forth, and from side to side to find equilibrium.

Sitting basic position:

Sit far out on the chair, on your sit bones (alternatively on the floor in meditation position with your legs crossed) with your feet firm in the ground. The back is erect and straight. Have an open feeling in the chest, guide your sternum slightly forward and upward to get your shoulders into place. Your chin is slightly pulled in to have your neck become an extension of the spine. Place your hand in the other, right hand in left, slightly below the navel.

Continuation for both standing and sitting:

Then close the eyes (alternatively fix your eyes at a point on the ground) and turn your focus inwards. Relax your thoughts and rest in yourself. Be aware of your breathing and take some deep breaths. Guide your breath to your lower belly and let your mind sink down to your center in Dan Tian, behind and below the navel. Let the mind rest in your breathing. Put the tip of your tongue to the palate, slightly behind your teeth, where the gum becomes a bit softer, and relax your jaw. Push upwards with your tongue 3 times. Keeping the tongue there throughout all of the exercises is recommended.

Move your attention down to your tailbone. Then move your focus up the spine, vertebra after vertebra, up to the neck and the base of the skull and lengthen your spine from within. Feel the ascending, upright force. The one that wants to be awake and alert. Be aware of and touch the space or sky above you. Then receive the descending force, the relaxation, the gravitational pull. Relax your face, around your eyes, behind your eyes and in your jaw. Shoulders and chest relax. The back, abdomen and legs relax. Then feel how your feet touch the ground and earth below.

Physical warm-ups exercises

Here are some warm-up exercises that help you loosen up your body before an exercise, one standing, one sitting and one lying version. With a relaxed lower abdomen and an erect and agile spine, the energy can travel more easily up from the pelvic floor to the brain. A Taoist saying goes: "You will not get any older than your spine is flexible".

Guide exercise 2:

Time: 10 min standing, 5 min sitting, 5 min lying

Purpose: Loosen up and relax your body ❤ Open up the spine ❤ Increase the Qi flow in your body

Preparation: Standing or sitting basic position.

Standing warm-up:

- Shake: Feel the connection to Mother Earth and let a shaking motion rise up from the ground and bounce up and down from the feet, then from the knees and then from the hips. Shake your shoulders, arms and wrists each in turn a little extra. Shake your head and then your chest, belly and buttocks. Finally shake the entire body. Stop abruptly and stand still for a while and experience your body.

- Open the hips and chest: tilt your pelvis backward by pulling in your tailbone between the legs. Then tilt your pelvis foreward, pull the tailbone backwards and arch your lower back as much as you can. Wiggle back and forth 10 times. Then circle 5 turns in each direction, successively, your tailbone, the entire pelvis and your chest.

- Spinal cord breathing: bend your arms with your hands in front of your chest. Make soft fists. Breathe in and open your chest and squeeze your shoulder blades by bringing your arms back and shoulder blades together and down, arch your back forward at the same time, like a duck tail. Breathe out, pull the tailbone in between your legs and arch back, the head hangs down slightly and the arms come together in front of the body. Do this 5 times.

Sitting warm-up:

- Lean your body forward from your hips down as far as it goes, until your stomach touches your knees. Roll up vertebra after vertebra, the neck and head comes up last. Do this 5 times.

- Roll down your chin first, then down vertebra after vertebra. Roll the body upwards from the hip. Do this 5 times.

- Rock your hip bones from side to side for a minute.

Lying warm-up:

- Lie on your back with your knees towards the ceiling and your feet on the floor. Rock the pelvis rhythmically back and forth, by moving your tailbone up and down, and let the movement develop through the spine all the way up to the neck. Rock 50 times.

- Lie on your back with stretched legs. Breathe in and tighten your fists and bend your ankles and push your toes upwards as much as you can. Hold your breath and imagine that you're pushing energy up through your body. Exhale and relax and guide the energy down the spine and down your legs. Do this 3 times.

- Breathe in and fill your chest with air. Hold your breath and push the air down to the abdominal area and then back into the chest. Press the air up and down 5 times. Exhale and relax. This provides a massage beneficial for the organs of the abdomen.

- Do the same thing again but now you breathe in and fill your abdominal area with air first. Hold your breath and push the air up into the chest and then back down into the abdomen again. Press the air up and down 5 times. Breathe out and relax.

Finishing up, collecting energy and yin phase

After the exercises that follow, it's important to preserve the energy: the Qi you have generated. You do this by focusing on and laying your hands on Dan Tian. Dan Tian is a neutral place where you can collect the energy, ground your experiences and cultivate your observational ability. The body is given the opportunity to digest the impressions and integrate the exercise. The energy movement that has begun is allowed to be completed. Feel the pulsation of the electromagnetic power. Allow yourself to listen with all your senses and be receptive and sensitive to all the sensations that arise. Going inside awakens the deeper wisdom of your body consciousness. The exercises also end with a so-called yin phase, where you only rest, observe and do nothing. Like meditation in silence, stillness and presence. It's in silence that you can be receptive and listen for answers and hear what you never heard before. The yin phase is important for the balance between activity and receptivity.

Guide exercise 3:

Time: 5 min

Purpose: Deposit energy into your energy account ❤ Ground your experience ❤ Nurture the development of your Dan Tian

Gather energy and yin phase:

❧ Put your hands on Dan Tian, just below the navel. Let your attention sink down there and collect the energy. Rest and yin phase. Do nothing, observe, integrate.

If you want to strengthen the gathering effect further, put your right hand on the navel and your left hand over the right. Circle your hands counterclockwise ten turns around the navel, small circles that grow bigger and bigger. Then ten circles clockwise, which become smaller and smaller.

The tree, exercise for grounding and inner power

This exercise develops your inner strength and gives you a more stable and open body. It helps you to ground yourself in your body and to become more centered and balanced. At a physical level you exercise relaxation, bodily awareness and a good posture. The mind learns concentration and to be more present. The more stable the body, the more energy you can cope with. The more relaxed the body is, the more calm and relaxed mind. The more open the body is, the more flow. This you will quickly notice if you practice regularly. Your body is waiting for you to move in fully and comletely and to be embodied and illuminated by your consciousness.

For devoted Qigong practitioners, there is nothing more exciting than standing still like a tree and observing how the mind behaves facing a feeling or pain. Being able to ”sneak up” on yourself and become completely blessed when a tension somewhere in the body will make itself noticed, resolve itself and release its energy. This process will end up being a fascinating adventure in your own bodily consciousness.

Perineum and crown

The point in the perineum is called Hui Yin the “Gate of Life and Death” and is situated between the bottom part of the vagina and the anus. It is a gathering place for yin energies. Through this gate, life energy can easily leak out. You can also let nourishing energy come in from Mother Earth and nurture you.

The crown is called Bai Hui, the point of “Hundred Convergences” and is situated on the top of the head, straight up from the ears. It is linked to the pineal gland and from here you can see the higher perspective and get in touch with Father Sky.

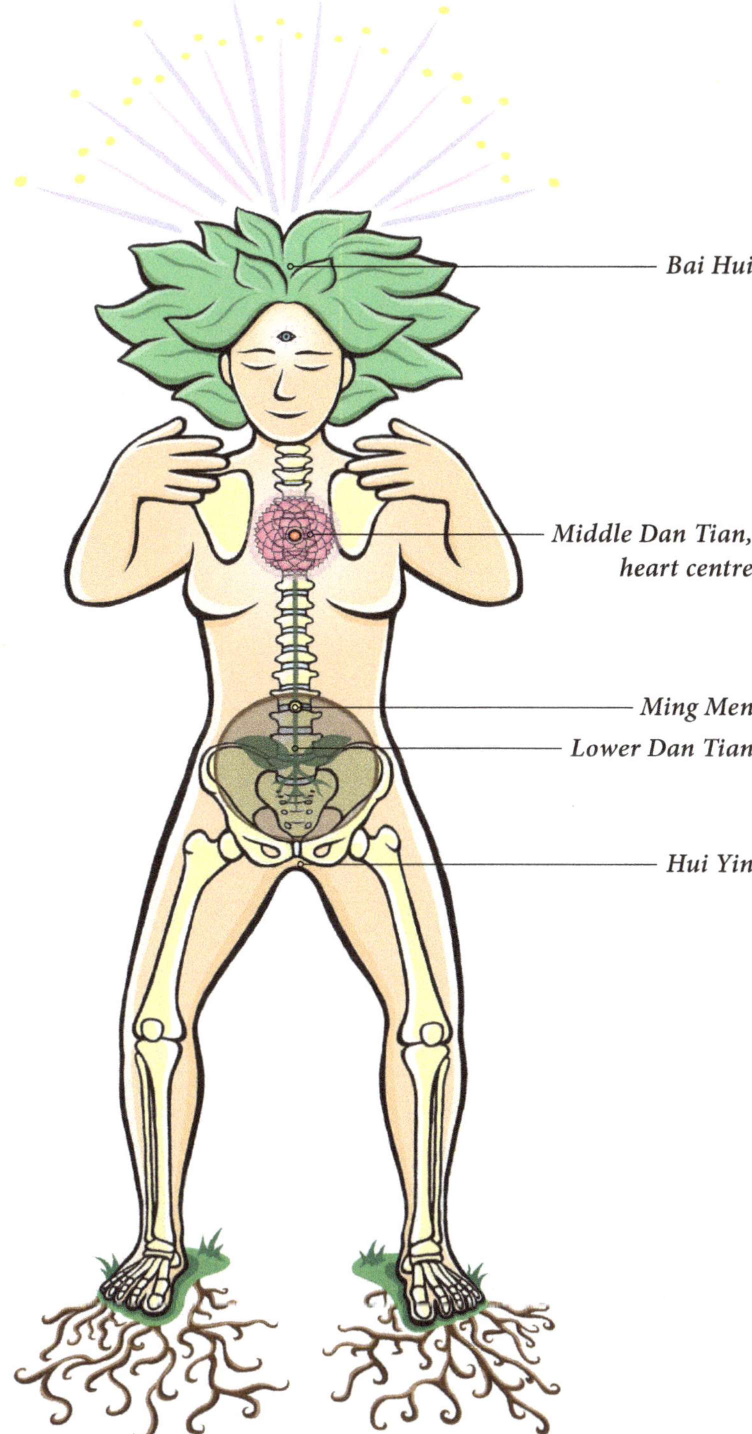

Imagine standing steady like a tree growing towards the light, with your roots deep down in the earth. You receive energy from the sun and nourishment from the earth. Feel the connection to both heaven and earth, while being aware of your own center, Dan Tian.

Guide exercise 4:

Time: 5-15 min

Purpose: To build a stable foundation and ground yourself in the body ❤ Open up to your inner power ❤ Balance yin and yang (heaven and earth)

Preparation: Standing basic position and warm-up exercises.

1. Stand in basic position. Bring your hands up at the heigth of your neck. Your arms are smoothly rounded as if you were hugging a tree. Your palms are facing you. Slightly spread your fingers. The little fingers point down and towards you and your thumbs up and away from you.

2. Relax the abdomen and buttocks. Imagine grabbing the ground a little extra with your toes. Let roots grow down into the earth, send your consciousness deep down and ground yourself in Mother Earth. Then feel the connection between your perineum and the earth. Be aware of the crown, the top of the head. Connect with the sky and draw the essence of the sun into your heart.

3. Turn your attention and all your senses inwards (see, listen, smell, feel, touch your inside). Relax your mind and breathe calmly and deeply. Guide your consciousness around within your body. Be aware of unnecessary tension anywhere. Strive to release tensions and open up inside. Correct your posture to basic position from time to time. Observe thoughts, feelings and body sensations that come and go. Perhaps pain and discomfort transforming into relaxation and pleasure. The aim is to relax more and more while being stable and standing straight.

4. Finish. Put your hands on Dan Tian, move your focus there and collect the energy. Rest and yin phase.

Begin by standing 5 minutes at each time. Increase gradually to 15 minutes. It's recommended to have a mirror to peek at sometimes to correct your posture.

The inner smile

This is one of the classic Taoist meditations. In this exercise, you smile in towards yourself and to your internal organs. In this way you activate a pleasant energy which you can consciously direct to different parts of your body. The meditation also develops a sense of acceptance and self-love. It is a deep recgnition that there is always an inner smile present, a deep sense of profound inner love. This is a yin opening, where you allow full self-acceptance of all of yourself, and allow yourself to be nourished and rejuvenated.

Andrew Fretwell's take on the inner smile:

Only our essence remains stable at all times. It is a neutral force we all have at our core. The inner smile is the conscious recognition and allowance of this. The inner smile is not something you do, but rather the recognition that at the core of every human being there's a self, that has never been traumatized, and is always free, like an inner sun that is always shining. It's a deep recognition of what is truth. Smiling this deep essence into our body over time gradually releases all unbalances out of our body. We need to address this at the physical dimension of ourselves and it is so much more powerful than meditation alone.

Center of well-being

All 108 muscles of the face are mapped and researchers have come to the conclusion that just by activating the muscles that raise the corners of your mouth and the laughing muscles around the eyes, you affect one of the centers of well-being in the brain, whether you're happy or not. The latest research on the brain and meditation also confirms that we can control our brain activity, and thereby reduce stress and increase well-being. One of the world's leading research scientists, David Richardson, has shown that the brain and our consciousness are way more plastic than we previously believed and can change using different techniques and meditation.

The intelligence of the heart

Research has also shown how emotions affect the biochemistry of the body. At the HeartMath Institute in California, they have tried to prove the intelligence of the heart, a fact that many aboriginal cultures have long been pointing out. Among other things, they have seen that, by shifting our focus from head to heart, we can change our attitude and increase the flow of well-being hormones and reduce stress hormones radically. The electromagnetic field of the heart is much stronger than the brain.

See if it works for you by looking at a conflict you have in your life, on the inside or something that's currently being played out in your relationships, on the outside. Consider the conflict from the two different perspectives. First from the perspective of the head, the center of reason and then from the heart, the center of compassion. How does your view and attitude to the conflict change? How does your feeling towards it change? Many people think this sounds way too simple to be true. Try and see if it works for you.

The internal organs

In Chinese medicine our emotional life and inner organs are connected. The organs in the abdomen have a consciousness and that is where you create and store your feelings. Feelings that you don't want to feel for various reasons do not disappear, but tend to stay inside of you. The energy stagnates and the body becomes tense. Like the food we eat, different experiences need to be digested and processed and we need to learn how to handle all the emotional expressions of being human.

Each yin organ (heart, spleen, lungs, kidneys, liver) has an associated yang organ (small intestine, stomach, large intestine, bladder, gallbladder). If an organ is weak, you may get stuck in a negative emotion, and on the contrary, a recurring negative emotion drains the organ. By incorporating a positive feeling, you can strengthen the organ. Courage and self-esteem, for example, strengthen the lungs and playfulness is good for the heart. A state of stress in the kidneys can be transformed into care and wisdom. Worry in the spleen turns into trust. However, we need all the human emotional expressions, both negative and positive. Feelings of fear help you to be alert in the face of danger, anger makes you able to set boundaries etc. According to Tao, it is as unhealthy to only feel kindness as it is to never feel grief.

In traditional Chinese medicine, the five element theory is used to diagnose and describe symptoms and conditions. Water, fire, metal, earth and wood represent different aspects and characteristics in us and are associated with different organs and senses. Tao believes that all aspects of life can be reflected in the elements. Going out and reflecting on yourself in nature is very relaxing and strengthening. A hike in the woods, resting on Mother Earth or on a mountain cliff, listening to a waterfall or looking into a fire. Among the most important things we can do is to create an elemental and emotional balance in our lives. In the chart below you can read about how elements, organs, feelings, expressions, colors and senses are connected. You can use the feeling and color of the organ to enhance the effect of your meditation. Stay a minute inside each organ. By helping the internal organs to relax, you balance your emotions.

The organs and the five element theory

Organ	Kidneys (bladder)	Heart (small intestine)	Lungs (large intestine)	Spleen (stomach, pancreas)	Liver (gall bladder)
Element	water	fire	metal	earth	wood
Color	blue	red	white	yellow	green
Negative emotion	fear, stress	malice, arrogance, impatience	sadness, depression, grief	mental worry, stress	anger, aggression, frustration
Positive emotion	caution, awareness, wisdom, stillness	love, playfulness, joy, enthusiasm	strength, courage, integrity, independence	stability, centering, compassion	kindness, generosity
Expression	life-force and the desire to live	to be able to give and receive	ability to let go and devote yourself	to have trust and a relaxed mind	will power, making decisions, creativity, expansion
Physical	regulate bodily fluids and blood pressure, purify the blood	pumps the blood	inhaling oxygene and exhaling carbomonoxid	filters the blood, supports immune system	assimilating nutrition and detoxing the blood
Position	by the lower back, close to the spine	in the chest, slightly to the left	in the chest	below the ribs to the left	partly below the ribs to the right
Sense	ears, hearing	tongue, speech	nose, smell	lips, taste	eyes, vision

Time: 10 min

Purpose: Transform negative energy into vitality ❤ Balance your organs and feelings ❤ Create an accepting inner atmosphere

Preparation: Sitting basic position.

1. Start out with a smile on your lips. Think of someone you like, a child, an animal, a place, something that really makes you smile. Then let go of the image and direct the smile inwards.

2. Direct your attention and smile at your heart. Guide your breath there and really feel the connection and awaken the energy. Feel, look into and listen to your heart. Maybe your heart smiles back at you. Feel happiness and playfulness and fill the heart with a red light.

3. Then move your attention to the spleen. Smile down at your spleen and guide your breath to touch it. Let the mind relax. Feel a sense of trust and fill the spleen with a yellow light.

4. Then move your attention to the lungs. Smile at them and guide your breath and your consciousness there. Feel a sense of self-esteem, courage and strength. Breathe in a white light into the lungs.

5. Then move your attention and smile at your kidneys. Breathe down into the kidneys. How are your kidneys doing? Feel and listen to them. Get them to relax. Feel stillness and be aware and alert. Let the kidneys bathe in a blue light.

6. Now move your attention to the liver and direct a smile there. Guide your breath there, watch and listen. Feel a sense of kindness and generosity. Allow the liver to be filled with green light.

7. Finally move the attention and the smile back to your heart. Collect happiness from the heart, trust from the spleen, courage from the lungs, stillness from the kidneys, generosity from the liver. Let everything gather in your heart.

8. These emotions and good vibrations are allowed to radiate and spread throughout the body and fill all your cells.

9. Finish. Put your hands on Dan Tian, move your focus there and collect the energy. Rest and yin phase.

The order follows the positive cycle of the five element theory of traditional Chinese medicine, where the elements support and nurture each other. The fire gives nutrition (ashes) to the earth, the earth produces metal, metal gives nutrients (minerals) to the water, the water nurtures the tree, and wood gives fuel to the fire. Examples of this negative cycle is metal that cuts down the tree or water that extinguishes the fire. Usually, only the nurturing cycle is used for internal exercises (see picture on p. 26).

The inner organs

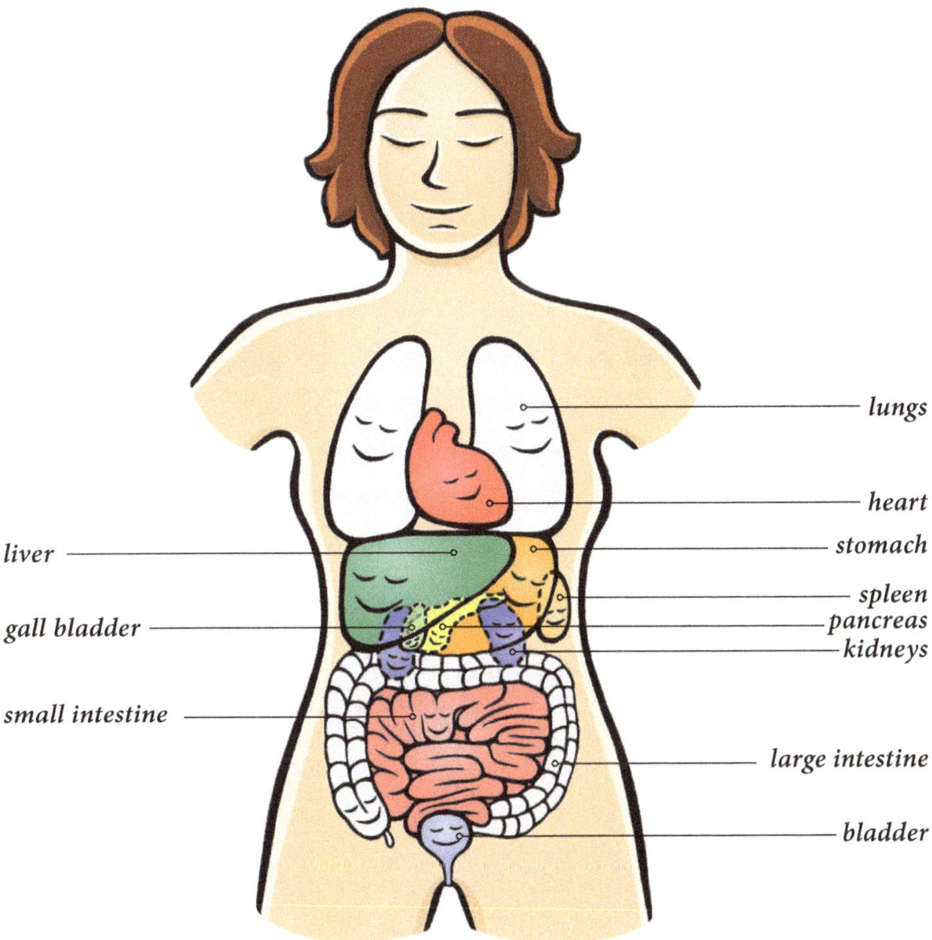

In Chinese medicine emotions and organs are connected. The organs have a consciousness and are where feelings are created and stored. By helping the organs relax you're making them happy and support your emotional balance

The short inner smile

Feel free to do this shorter version before other exercises in connection with the basic positions. It will put you in a state of deeper presence and a positive atmosphere. It's a simple, effective and soothing exercise that you can, in principle, perform anywhere and at any time.

Guide Exercise 6:

Time: 5 min

Purpose: Turn your focus inwards ❤ Create a state of presence ❤ Develop an attentive and peaceful attitude

Preparation: Sitting or standing basic position.

1. Start out with a smile on your lips. Think of someone you like, a child, an animal, a place, something that really makes you smile. Then let go of the image and direct the smile inwards.

2. Direct your attention and smile at your heart. Guide your breath there and really feel the connection and awaken the energy. Fall into the void of your heart. Feel, look into and listen to your heart.

3. From there drop down your awareness into your center. Smile down at Dan Tian and the lower abdomen. Feel the electromagnetic power pulsate within you.

4. Then smile down at your genitals. Feel and awaken subtle exited energy and let your life force expand.

5. Then guide the energy and the smile up the spine and through the nervous system throughout your body. Let the smile penetrate every cell and make them energized and happy.

6. Finish. Put your hands on Dan Tian and rest for a short while.

Now you are in a favorable state to move on to other exercises or take on everyday life.

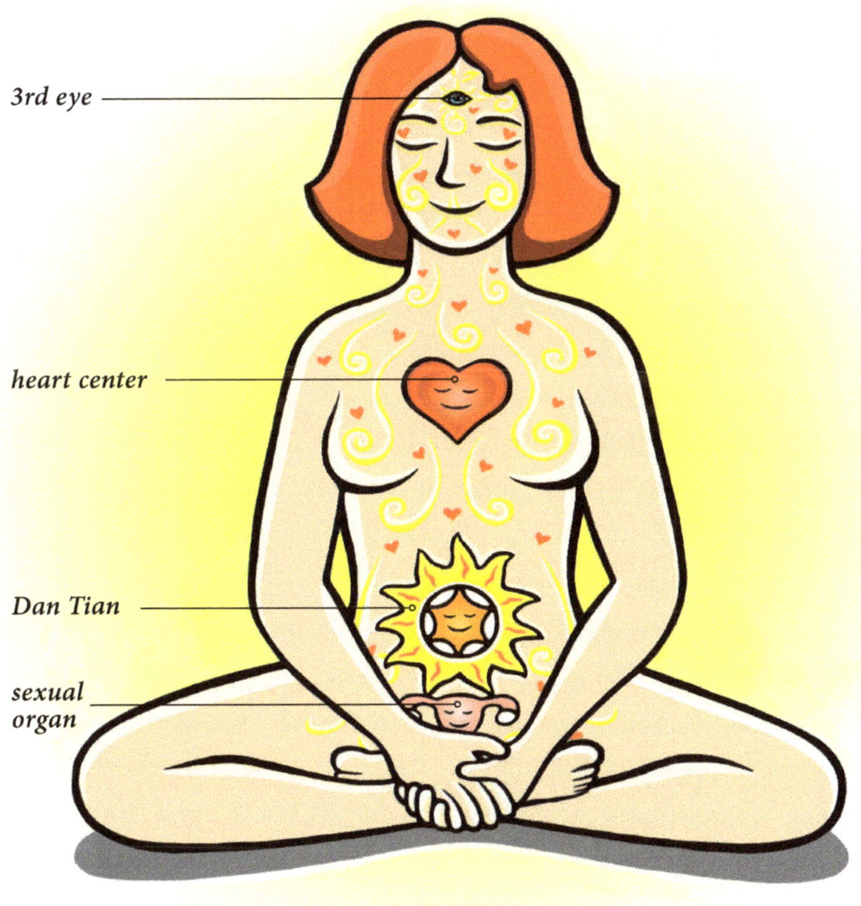

The inner smile creates a positive and loving inner atmosphere.

The small circulation

The small circulation (SC) is an exercise where you circulate, transform and distribute your energy. Being able to know and guide Qi through different centers and meridians in the body is the very foundation of Taoist energy work. In SC, the energy is circulated along the two central meridians, Du Mai (yang) that goes up the spine and down Ren Mai (yin) that goes down the front side of your body. The channels help to regulate the flow of yin and yang energy in the other 12 organ-related meridians. The Qi is then spread throughout the body. One purpose of Qigong is specifically to create a fresh energy flow for these "rivers" of Qi. Du Mai also supply Qi to the nervous system, the cells need to be nourished with Qi to function well. Circulating Qi in these channels is important to stay healthy. SC also links important energy points and energy centers. When Qi is allowed to flow freely in the SC, the entire body is nurtured and harmonized. The life energy is cleared and refined. You get a strong and resilient body and a clear and flexible mind. Work with this circulation is not only done within Tao but also in several other traditions.

Du Mai and Ren Mai

Du Mai starts in the perineum (between the bottom part of the vagina and anus) and goes up along the spine, to the base of the skull and the crown, and then down through the point between the eyebrows and ends in your palate. Ren Mai takes over the circulation down through the tongue and goes down the front side of your body and ends up in the perineum. You place the tip of your tongue up on the palate to tie the two meridians together and to ground the energy in your body. The channels run about a centimeter into the body. The points are inputs to energy centers in the body.

Taoist mystic says: *In the beginning there was only the void, WuJi, which holds the potential of all things. In the creation, when egg (yin) and sperm (yang) met and attached to the uterus wall, the attachment became Chi Hai (navel) and the opposite became Ming Men (lower back). From Chi Hai, Ren Mai (water) was created and from Ming Men, Du Mai (fire) was created and in the middle emerged the third channel Chong Mai. From this, the 10,000 things emerged.*

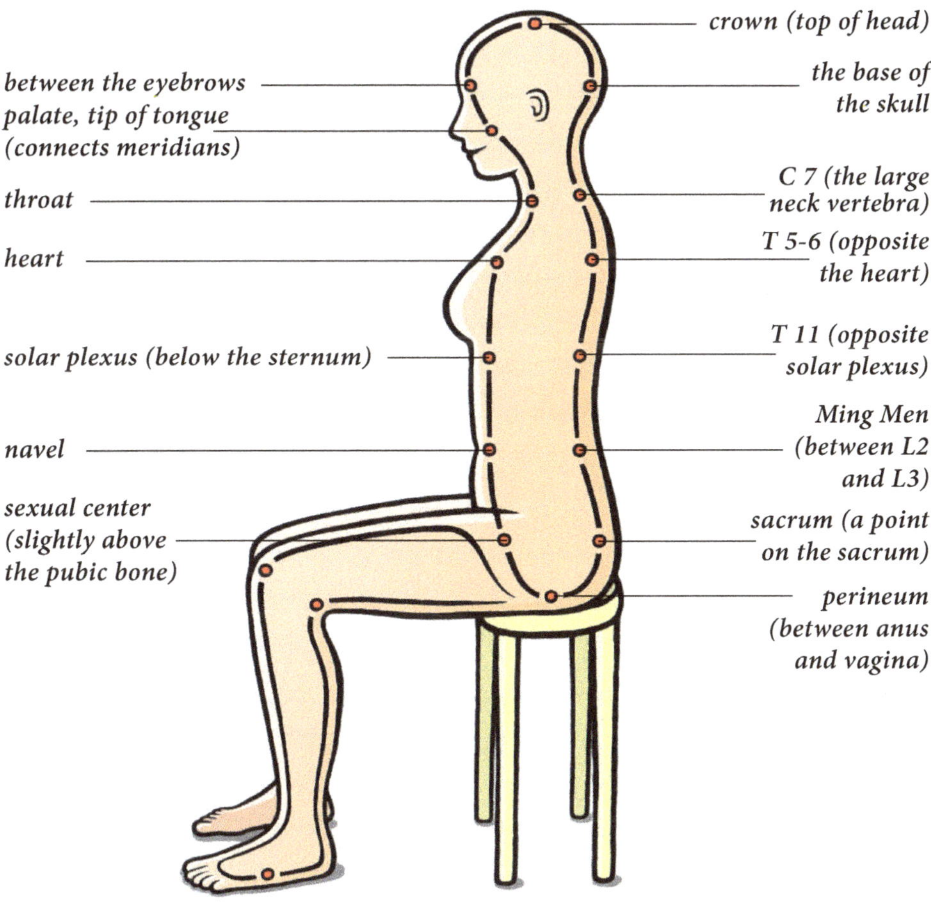

To open this circulation fully is a lifetime project with full enlightenment as a goal. So have perseverance and enjoy the work along the way.

Explore the points

You connect with and open the points by directing your attention and a smile to each point. Breathe in and out through the point. Also strengthen the connection with the help of a clear focus and using your inner eyes and ears. Be present and let your awareness touch every point. Feel how the points open up and relax. Experience, explore and perceive each point. Does it feel relaxed or blocked? How is it to focus on each point? Or looking out at the world or perceiving the world from there? Does it feel comfortable or unpleasant? Is there a lot of energy or a small amount of energy? Are there any distinctions between the different points?

Stay longer on the points in the back, preferably a few minutes on each. On the front side of your body, the energy flows like a waterfall and touches the points on the way down. The more the points open, the easier it becomes to circulate the energy in SC. Eventually you'll be able to do a whole round on one breath.

At first, it may be difficult to concentrate and feel the points. But it usually gets easier over time. One effect, and many agree with me, is that a nice feeling is created in the body as energy begins to flow and the mind becomes more peaceful, open and relaxed.

Through your mind you can lead Qi to any part of the body. You develop the sensitivity to feel each part of the body internally. Important is as well to really feel the Qi. The deeper the mind reaches in the meditations the more profound and beautiful these exercises will be. You can trust that your presence will make a difference.

Time: 15 min

Purpose: Circulate Qi and provide the body with life energy ❤ Open, activate and connect different energy centers in the body ❤ Unravel physical and mental blockages

Preparation: Sitting basic position, sitting warm-up and a short inner smile.

1. Focus and breath in Dan Tian. Go deep inside, behind and below the navel. Sink down into it.

2. Breathe in and imagine pulling the energy from Dan Tian down to the next point, the sexual center above the pubic bone. Breathe out through this point.

3. Breathe in and imagine pulling the energy down from the sexual center to the next point, perineum, between the anus and the bottom part of the vagina. Breathe out and stay in the perineum. Rest, explore and breathe in and out of the point in the perineum. Stay a few minutes in each point.

4. Then inhale through the perineum and guide the energy up to the next point, at the center of the sacrum. Breathe out and stay on this point. Rest, explore and breathe in and out through the sacrum.

5. Continue in the same way to move the energy up through the entire spine and go through each point. Ming Men, opposite the navel, T11, opposite solar plexus, T5, between the shoulder blades, C7, the neck, base of the skull and the crown, top of the head.

6. Then put the tip of the tongue on the palate and guide the energy faster down your front, between the eyebrows, through the tongue down to the throat, the heart point, solar plexus, the navel, the sexual center and finally the perineum. Rest in your perineum for a while.

7. Now breathe in and drag the energy through all the points, up the spine, hold your breath and keep your focus a few seconds in the crown. Then exhale, and let the energy flow down through the points on the front. Keep the tip of your tongue against your palate at all times.

8. Circle the energy 10 turns. One round per breath.

9. Finish. Put your hands on Dan Tian, keep your focus there and collect the energy. Rest and Yin phase.

Breast massage

The breasts are central to a woman's experience of ecstasy. They are directly connected to both the brain and the sex through the endocrine system and contain lots of smaller glands. Through stimulation, hormones that open up the vagina are secreted and increase your receptivity. The inner heart opens. Loving attention on the breasts and heart is usually the safest way to a woman's love, interest and devotion.

Massage your breasts frequently and with joy to stimulate circulation, sensitivity and self-love. Improvise and find out which sort of touch they appreciate the most. The breasts will then be happy and alive and filled with a positive aura. Regular massage can also prevent PMS and heavy menstrual periods. This exercise is sometimes called "The Deer Exercise".

Breast massage

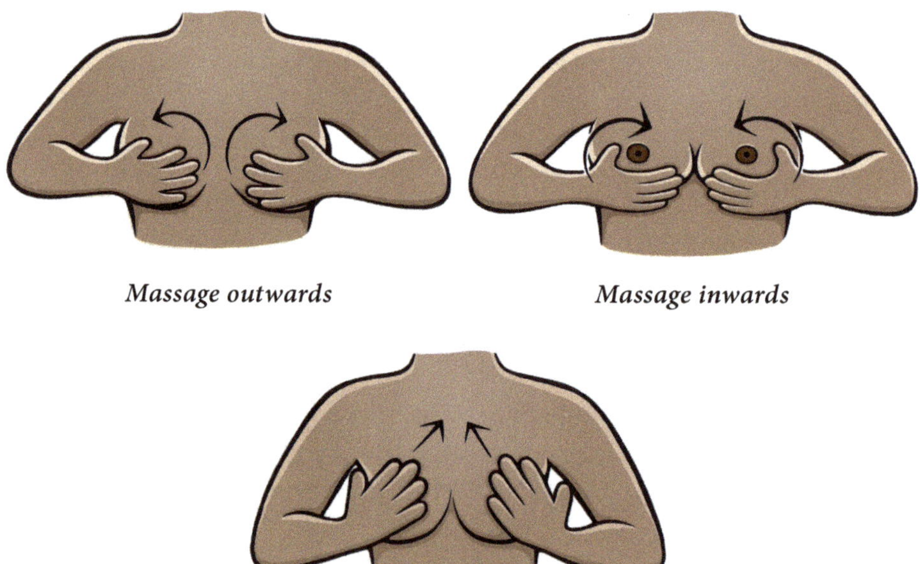

Connect with your breasts, how do they feel? The breasts are often used to being judged from the outside. Now feel them from the inside. Give them your attention, acceptance and gratitude for the joy and nourishment they give you.

Guide Exercise 8:

Time: 10 min

Purpose: Healthier and more sensitive breasts ❤ Increase circulation ❤ Give your breasts appreciation

Preparation: Sitting basic position.

1. Sit on a chair, or in meditation position with a heel against your genitals if you can.

2. Rub your hands warm.

3. Put your hands on your breasts.

4. Fill the breast with your presence, smile and breathe towards them and experience them from the inside.

5. Do 20 quick squeezes with the pelvic floor muscles.

6. Massage the breast 20 turns outwards (up the middle, out, down the sides) and then 20 turns inward (up the sides, in, down the middle).

7. Then place your hands on the outside of your breasts and push diagonally upwards, 20 times.

8. Place your fingers on your nipples and feel the connection to the ovaries. Guide the energy down to your genitals.

9. Sit still and feel the energy flow.

Charge your life energy

This exercise stimulates your breasts, kidneys and ovaries. The kidneys are placed quite high up in your lower back area, where the lumbar spine meets the thoracic spine, adjacent to and in front of the spine. To find the ovaries, put your thumbs in your navel and index fingers together just above the pubic bone. Where the little fingers end up is where the ovaries are.

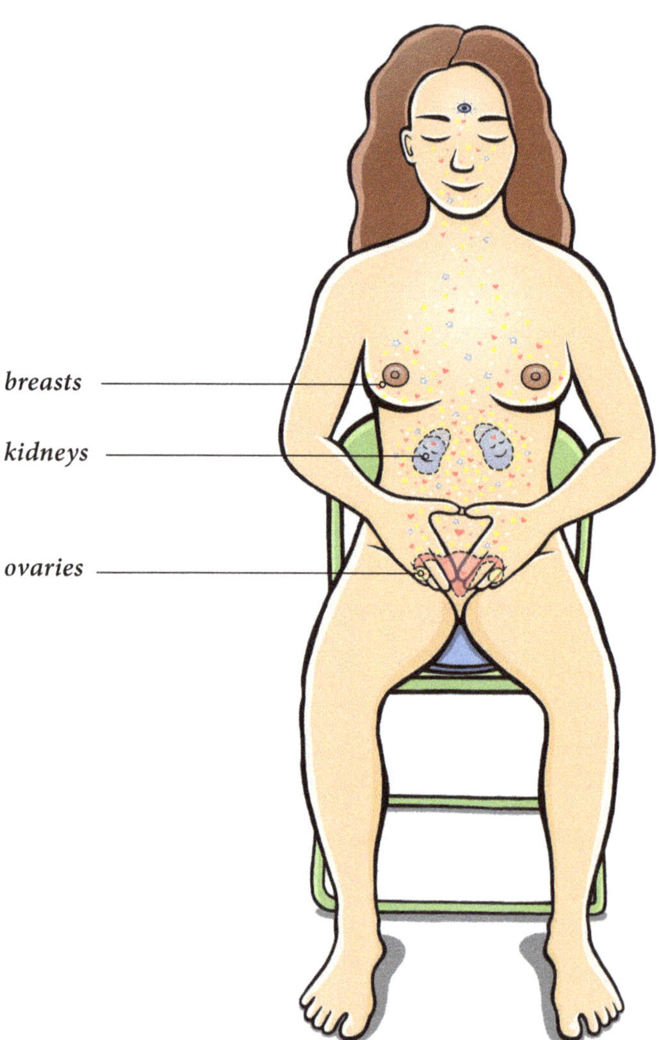

Guide exercise 9:

Time: 10 min

Purpose: Activate Dan Tian ❤ Connect the different parts ❤ Awaken energy

Preparation: Sitting basic position and a short inner smile.

1. Rub your hands warm.

2. Put your tongue up against the palate.

3. Put your hands on your breasts

4. Massage your breasts around the nipples with your whole hand. Start outwards 10 turns (up the center, down the sides). Pause, focus on your heart center.

5. Then massage your breasts inwards 10 turns (down the center, out, up the sides). Pause, focus on your heart center.

6. Move your hands to the kidneys.

7. Massage the kidneys. Rub with your fingers or the back of your hands up and down.

8. Pause, focus in Ming Men.

9. Massage the kidneys again. Pause, focus in Ming Men.

10. Place your hands on the ovaries - put your thumbs in your navel and index fingers together just above the pubic bone. Where the little fingers end up is where the ovaries are.

11. Massage the ovaries. Start outwards - from the pubic bone, up the center to navel, out, down along the groins. 10 turns.

12. Paus. Focus in the sexual center, just above the pubic bone.

13. Massage the ovaries. Inwards - from the pubic bone, up along the groins, into the navel, down to pubic bone. 10 turns.

14. Then hold your right thumb in your navel, your middle finger on your sexual center, slightly above the pubic bone, and the back of your left hand on Ming Men, your lower back. Focus in the middle of the triangle in your body.

15. Breathe into the three points, breathe out in the middle of the triangle, in Dan Tian. You do this to fill the Dan Tian with energy. Your uterus is a part of Dan Tian. Breathe calmly and deep for 10 breaths.

16. Continue with ovarian breathing and SC.

17. Or just finish and put your hands on Dan Tian, move your focus there and gather your energy. Rest and yin phase. Also, have a soft focus in your heart center.

EXERCISE 10:

Ovarian breathing

A woman has several hundred thousands of eggs in her ovaries. Each egg holds the potential to create life. The egg holds the essence of your vitality, your yin nature, your DNA and your Jing energy. To awaken and use this slumbering power Taoists created ovarian breathing. It stimulates the production of hormones and takes advantage of the essential energy of the eggs, and transforms it into life energy.

The activated potency of the eggs or the subtle, aroused energy is guided into the SC. The Jing energy needs to be circulated and refined to be used and to vitalize your body. Sexual energy is raw material that needs to be transformed. When the energy is transported through the spinal column it is refined and becomes more subtle and can then be used by the brain and taken care of by the body. This exercise is sometimes called the "fountain of youth" and has several favorable effects.

The essence of the eggs and aroused energy

In ovarian breathing, you are thereby taking advantage of the feminine essence of the eggs and subtly aroused energy. You can also progress with this exercise and train yourself with more aroused and orgasmic energy. Then it's important that the channels are open for the energy to move in the SC without excessive blockages. Once you have been training yourself, you can also proceed together with a partner. But it is by yourself you learn the most and where you train yourself, not in the heat of the moment. Eventually you'll learn how to focus the energy with only your intention, but until then, use the technique of training and guiding the energy. It will pay off.

Caress yourself

A good and energizing way to get to know and be intimate with your orgasmic energy is to self-pleasure. You can masturbate and caressing yourself as if you want to satisfy yourself. Focus at the same time on the perineum and continue until you almost have an orgasm. Relax and wait for a little while. Continue to touch yourself and focus on the cervix and the sexual center, at the height of the pubic bone. When you are almost there, you stop and wait again. Continue and do the same with focus on the navel and finally the heart, and then continue until you come. Then, sit still and observe the body sensations and where the orgasmic energy wants to go.

In this way you build the orgasmic energy. You will also train yourself to hold space for the sexual energy to find its way and move naturally around inside the body. Changing and varying your masturbation pattern is evolving and rewarding. Try out all your,

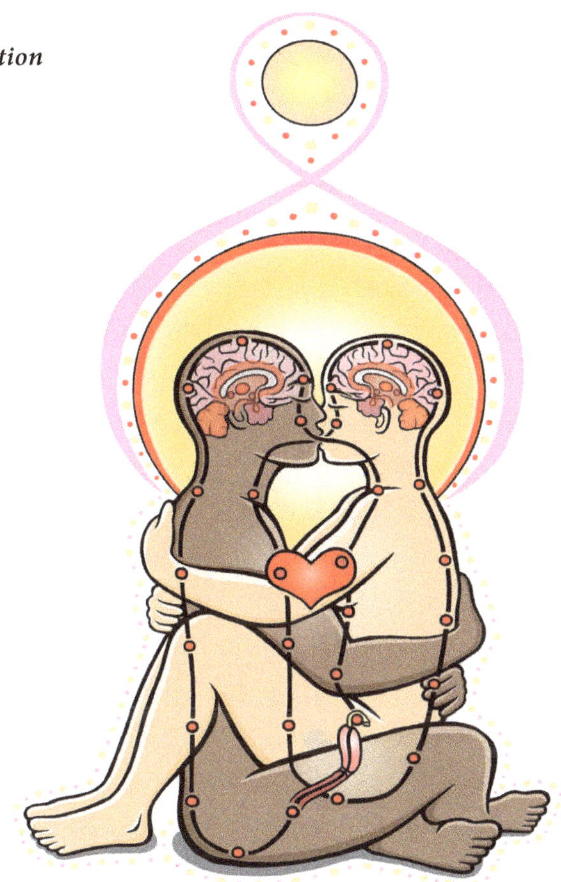

Cultivation with a partner and circulating the energy between each other.

maybe recently discovered, erotic body parts. I also recommend you to self-pleasure, regardless of being in a relationship or not.

Cultivation with partner

If you have a partner, you can circulate the energy into two circles that intersect. You receive the partner's energy through the tongue, guide it down your front and over to your partner again through your genitals. It then goes up your partner's spine and back to you. At the same time, your partner receives your energy through his tongue, and guides it down his front channel into your genitals and then the energy goes up through your spine again. The energy circulates as an eight between the two of you.

When is it best to perform ovarian breathing?

Ovarian breathing has the best effect on you when it is done in between your period and ovulation when the eggs are in the development phase and the energy is the strongest. If you are going through menopause, ovarian breathing is good at any time. According to Tao, there is still Jing energy in the ovaries which can be recovered as well as stimulating your libido. Some women experience their menopause issues decrease when they perform this exercise regularly.

Without uterus and ovaries

Even if you have had your ovaries or uterus removed, you can do these exercises. The energy imprint and the sensations are still there. It is worth taking care of the area where the organs were situated and to give it extra attention, love and acceptance. It will support and increase circulation and restore a healthy energy flow. Also the egg exercises further in are helpful, as it is particularly important to strengthen the pelvic floor muscles to assist the abdominal organs, and prevent them from "falling" down, especially if the uterus has been removed.

How the ability to have an orgasm is affected depends largely on how nerves and blood vessels are affected during surgery. The vaginal pleasure is more often influenced because it is linked to the pelvic nerve, which is connected to the uterus, while the pudendal nerve, which is associated with the clitoris, remains intact.

Other genital issues

If you have other problems in your genital area, such as vestibulitis, vaginismus, endometriosis, myoma, cysts, inflammation or urinary tract infections, perform the exercise softly and focus on sensitivity and on deepening the connection to your genitals. It's not the exercise in itself that will heal you, but your presence, acceptance and intention. Take into account the placebo effect, cell regeneration, body awareness and the power of the mind to influence your biochemistry when you perform the practices. The exercises are tools that help and guide you along the way. The body speaks to us in many different ways. Insight into the how's and the why's comes through deep self-knowledge, in all aspects; physically, emotionally, mentally, spiritually and sexually. Everything is connected and interacts intimately.

Conventional medical care or alternative treatments should of course be used when needed.

My own experience of healing magic

I managed to heal myself from a tumor in one of my ovaries. It was a tumor of the kind that should be operated on as soon as possible or as the doctor expressed it: "If you were my wife I would perform the surgery on you tomorrow morning". I was obviously scared and unsure of what I should do. What was crucial was that I did not feel sick, had no symptoms and therefore it felt absurd that they were going to go inside me to dig around. That's why I quickly made the decision to first do what I could myself. After years of Qigong training and accompanied bodily awareness, I felt quite confident in going with my instincts. Beside deepening these Taoist exercises, I spent a few years trying everything from homeopathy, to herbs, to shamanic healing. Therefore, it's hard to point out exactly what made me whole again. In any case, the tumor is now gone, and is according to the medical professionals completely inexplicable. An important part of the healing was a deeper understanding of myself as a woman and how I use my creative force in life. It is my conviction that the different symptoms of the body are it's way to speak to us and point to unconscious patterns that long for full freedom.

Abuse

If you have been subjected to abuse, be it physically or mentally, the communication and connection with your womb may have been broken. In addition, we often accuse ourselves of what occurred and add yet another repulsive emotion to the unpleasantries that have already happened. The keys to healing can be forgiveness, embracing your womb, reconnecting with your feelings, and understanding how your mind works and thereby freeing yourself from guilt and shame. Your inner guide and your soul force can turn trauma into wisdom. If you have unmanageable or recurring destructive thoughts and feelings about this, seek professional help. Being mirrored by a neutral and professional person can be illuminating and of great value.

Note!

If you are worried or stressed, make sure you have the ability to ground yourself before you do the ovarian breathing. If you are pregnant do not do the exercise. If you want to get pregnant, do the exercise softly and easily.

Guide exercise 10:

Time: 15 min

Purpose: Refine, transform and guide the sexual energy, Jing Qi ❤ Train yourself to bring energy up along your spine ❤ Nurture the hormone system, nervous system and the brain

Preparation: Breast massage or charge your life energy to activate your sexual energy.

1. Direct your attention towards your genitals, especially the ovaries.

2. Breathe in and squeeze the pelvic floor muscles softly and feel the ovaries as you squeeze. Breathe out into the ovaries and relax. Keep breathing in this way until the area is filled with a warm nice pleasurable feeling. Note which sort of squeeze activates the most energy - hard, soft, light, sucking, sensual, fast. Learn more about various ways of squeezing on p. 131.

3. Now you should guide the energy from the perineum to different points in your back. You do this by simultaneously squeezing, inhaling and pulling the energy up from the perineum to the next point. Then breathe out into that point, relax and fill it with the energy. Go straight back to the perineum again and breathe in, squeeze and move the energy up. Do about 3-5 pulls to each point. Or continue until the point is filled.

4. The first point you guide the energy to is the sacrum. Continue to T11, then C7, the base of the skull and the crown. You draw the energy all the way from the perineum and up the spine to the respective point, in one breath and one squeeze. Breathe out into the point.

5. After filling the crown you breathe in and hold your breath and keep your attention there and then circulate the energy just above the crown 3-5 times counterclockwise, and then again clockwise. Let your inner eyes "look around" the crown point in your inner world.

6. Then breathe out and let the energy flow down like a waterfall on the front side of your body along the frontal meridian, point by point, but now faster. The tongue is up against your palate.

7. Then circulate the energy in SC. First, you can go one turn, point by point and now also include Ming Men and the back of the heart point, T5. Then you can pull the energy around on one breath. Let the energy circle 10 turns.

8. Finish. Put your hands on Dan Tian, move your focus there and collect the energy. Rest and yin phase. Have a soft focus in your heart center.

You can do this exercises with a soft and subtle focus, like a light breeze is moving up the spine, or more powerful, with vigorous squeezes and breath and movement in your hips.

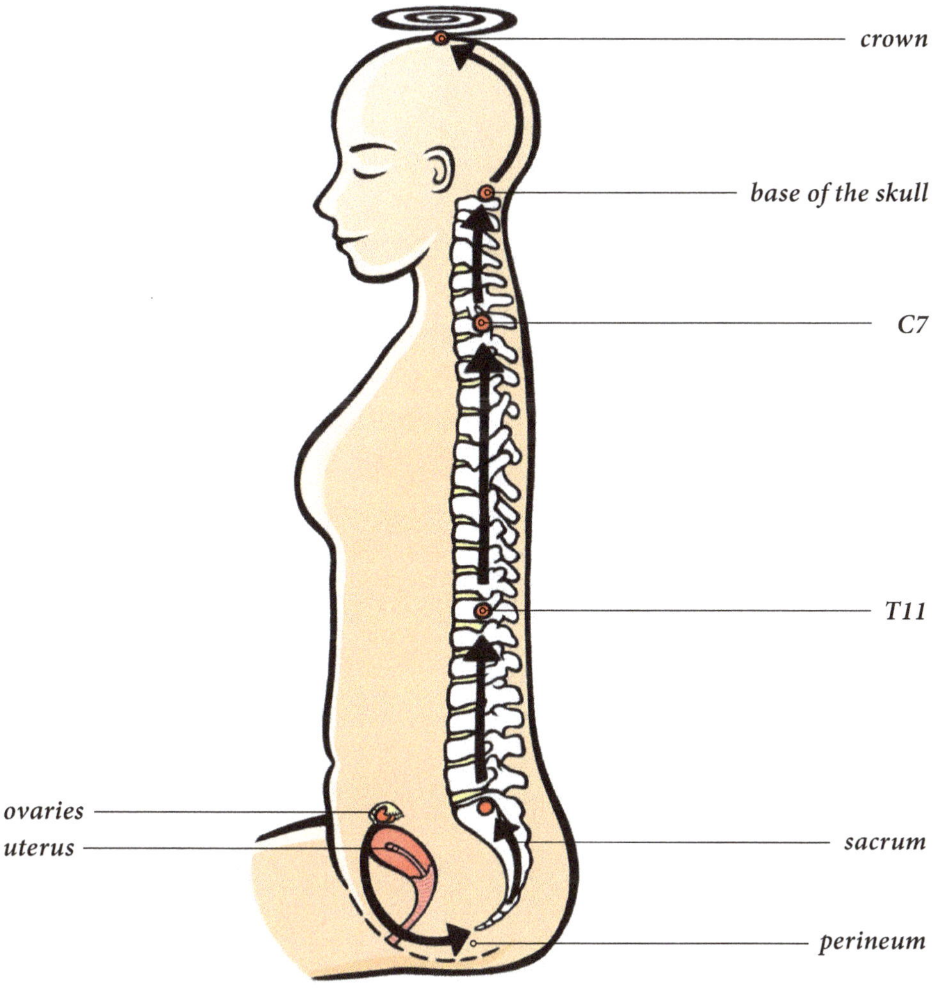

In ovarian breathing you work on lifting and guiding the energy up along the spine.

EXERCISE 11:

Hormone shower

The word hormone means "to awaken to life" or movement. The endocrine glands produce these chemical substances, which transmit signals through the blood to the different parts of the body. The body produces many different kinds of hormones and many are still being discovered. Hormones affect multiple functions, including blood pressure, metabolism, genital functions, blood sugar levels and energy supply.

The different glands interact in a very elegant and sensible manner and the hormone system is extremely important and central to our well-being. Therefore, you always go through all the glands when doing this exercise. It is also very important to rest afterwards and to allow the body to integrate. It is a very strong and rejuvenating exercise. The endocrine system is also very sensitive to stress and an unbalance can decrease your libido. This exercise will help you to recover from too much stress and restore vitality. I cannot emphasize enough the importance of the yin phase to take advantage of the peace afterwards.

The thrusting channel

The thrusting channel, Chong Mai, travels like a pipe through the core of the body. From the perineum through the cervix and all the way up to the brain. Along the way, the canal affects the glands and thus the chakras, the energy centers in the body. The channel absorbs and projects energy and it is through the energy centers that we experience and meet the world. These need to be open but also in contact with each other for a full life experience. This channel is a key to great transformation and awakenings to spiritual realms. Working with this channel will nourish health and will help to balance your emotions.

The gate of origin

The mouth of the cervix is an important point called Guan Yuan, which means "gate of origin". It's much like a gate you can go in or out through. Usually it opens outwards during menstruation and childbirth. During orgasm, it opens up inwards. Therefore, women, unlike men, do not lose energy during the orgasm. You open this door symbolically in the exercise hormone shower. You may view it as exploring the origin of life. By performing this exercise you fill up the supplies of your primordial life force energy.

The glands are entrances to other worlds

Each gland can be attributed to different qualities besides hormone production. The gland can be seen as a gateway to another reality. By strengthening your connection to the glands, their dormant forces can be aroused and become guides to deeply transforming experiences. The glands correspond with the points you open in the small circulation. Balancing and raising the energy levels in the glands is an important part of the Taoist way of developing, healing and strengthening the physical body as well as balancing the emotions. When the energy is transformed, a sort of vitality is produced which radiates from all of you, and is very invigorating and refreshing. The different characteristics of the glands are described below, as are their basic functions and hormone productions. Then two exercises follow to increase your connection to the glands, as well as the equilibrium of the endocrine system. Read more about hormones and their properties in the hormone glossary at the end of the book (p. 141-144).

The pineal gland: The mother of spirit

Attributes: Pineal gland, or the "soul's dwelling" as it is also called, helps you to get in touch with the spiritual, to surrender to the greater consciousness. It's like an antenna, it can send and receive messages. Guiding you to the light. Controls the other glands.
Physical function: Controls cycles, day rhythm and perception of light through eyes and skin.
Hormones: Oxytocin, serotonin, melatonin, DMT.
Located: Large as half of a pea and situated on the roof of the middle brain, located at the rear edge of the third ventricle and attached to the thalamus.

The pituitary gland: The mother of intelligence

Attributes: Helps you develop your psyche and your independence. The way to wisdom and the memory of who you are. Vision, compassion, devotion.
Physical function: Regulates growth, water and mineral balance. Managing director of the other glands.
Hormone: Oxytocin, prolactin. Luteinizing (LH) and follicle-stimulating hormone (FHS) which controls the reproduction cycle and the secretion of sex hormones.
Located: Behind the point between the eyebrows, on a branch under the hypothalamus. About the size of a pea.

The thyroid gland: The mother of growth

Attributes: Supports you to continue searching, growing and developing. The gateway to your strength of mind and the experience of meaningfulness.
Physical function: Affects metabolism in all cells of the body and regulates body temperature. Four small parathyroids are located on the back of the thyroid and regulate calcium metabolism in your bones.
Hormone: Thyroxine (T3 and T4)
Located: In front of and on both sides of the trachea.

The thymus gland: The mother of heart

Attributes: Sometimes called the rejuvenation gland. Guides you to the highest form of love. Also teaches you about creativity, talents, beauty and harmony.

Physical function: The thymus is very important for the lymph and immune system. It's also active during the growth phase of puberty.

Hormone: Thymosin which support the formation of T-lymphocytes, white blood cells which work for the immune system.

Located: Behind the sternum just above the heart and is about 2x1,5x0,2 inches.

The pancreas: The mother of transformation

Attributes: Supports transformation and integration of emotions. Guides you from your need of control to trust and compassion.

Physical function: Digestion, regulates sugar metabolism.

Hormone: Insulin and glucagon.

Located: Partially behind the stomach to the left, just below the ribs. It is elongated and about 5-6 inches long.

The adrenal glands: The mother of water and fire

Attributes: Provides nutrition and energy to your kidneys, genitals, bone marrow and your spine. Provides strength and awareness to both mental development and physical training.

Physical function: Associated with the nervous system, brain, bone marrow. The adrenal glands also produce substances that are vital to the body's metabolism of minerals, trace elements, carbohydrates, fat and protein.

Hormone: Produces the stress hormones cortisol and adrenaline and the feel good hormone DHEA and aldosterone, progesterone, estrogen and testosterone.

Located: The kidneys are approximately the size of your ears and the adrenals are located on top of them like small triangular hats. Situated close to the spine approximately between L1 and T11.

The ovaries: The mother of essence

Attributes: Provides vigor for your uterus, vagina, ovaries, breasts and sexuality.

Physical function: Produces eggs and female sex hormones. Important for genital development, cycles, heart and bone marrow.

Hormone: Estrogen, progesteron, DHEA, testosterone, relaxin.

Located: The size of an almond. If you place your thumbs in your belly button and your index fingers on the sexual center, your pinkies will end up above your ovaries.

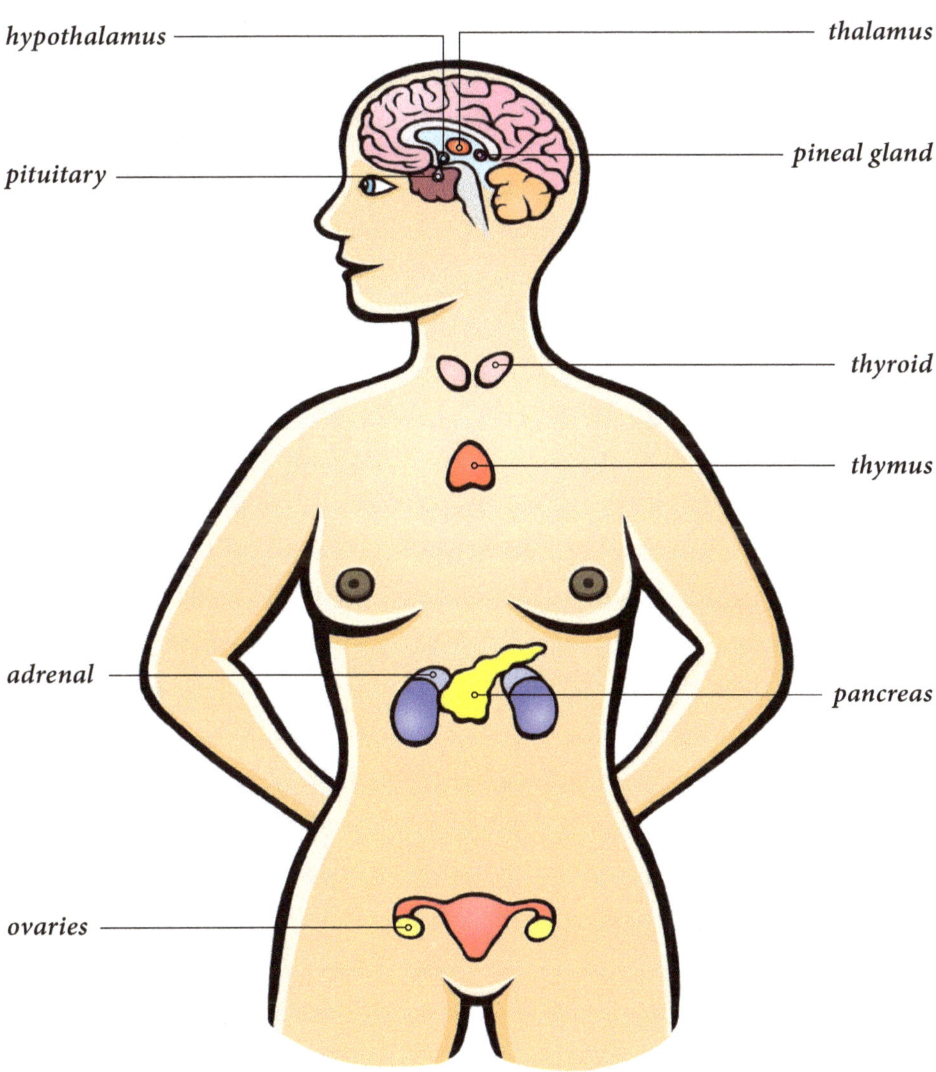

The endocrine glands can be attributed to different qualities and can be seen as entrances to other worlds. The awakening of the glands will increase your well-being and deepen your life experience.

Time: 30 min

Purpose: Connect to and explore the glands ❤ Balance the hormone system ❤ Bind the energy centers together

Preparation: Sitting basic position, warm-up exercises and a short inner smile.

1. Direct your attention to your pineal gland and stay there. Smile at the pineal gland to establish a connection. Let your breath, your presence and your consciousness touch the pineal gland. Look with your inner eyes, listen with your inner ears, and explore what it's like to be there. You might receive images, messages, a sensation or maybe you won't. It doesn't matter what happens, your presence will still affect and stimulate the area, as an inner subtle massage of your glands.

2. Continue to do the same thing with your pituitary, thyroid gland, thymus gland, pancreas, adrenal glands, and your ovaries. Stay for at least a few minutes on each gland.

3. As you have gone through all the glands, you move your focus to the perineum.

4. Breathe in and guide the energy up through the canal in the middle of the body, Chong Mai, the thrusting channel, which touches all glands and chakras on the way up.

5. Breathe out through the top of your head and let the energy spray all over like a fountain and shower yourself with this sparkling hormone energy. Go down to the perineum again and breath like this 3-6 times.

6. Then lay down and rest for 15 minutes.

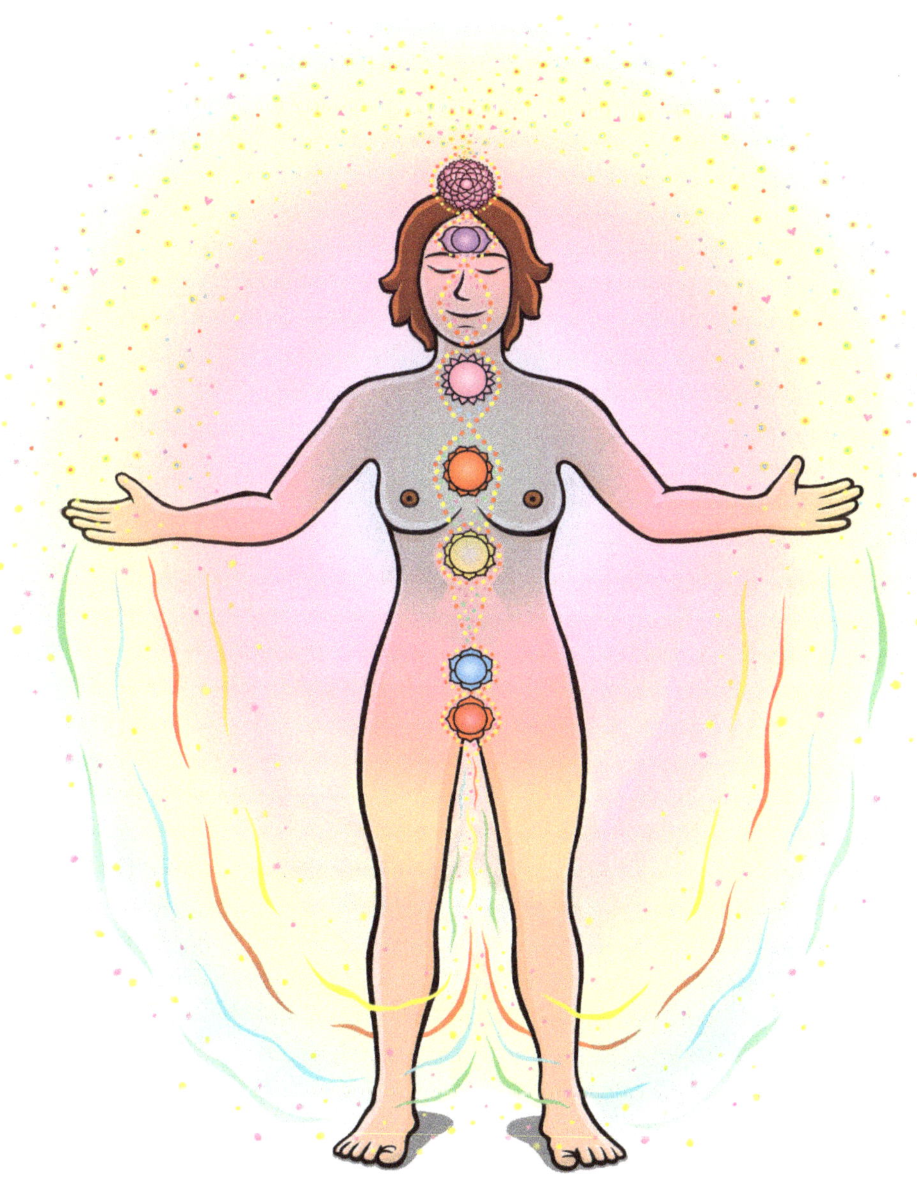

In the exercise Hormone shower, you are guiding the energy up through Chong Mai, which goes up the middle of your body and touches the glands and chakras.

Breast massage and gland exercise

Breast massage activates the sexual energy. When you massage your breasts, you become aware of the Qi that is activated and of how you open up to yourself. The nerves in the breasts and clitoris are linked to all major organs and glands, mainly through the vagus nerve. During this exercise you are combining the Jing-energy you activate in your breasts with the Jing-energy in the glands. This is where you connect the catalytic power with the energy of the hormone system - both are related to your essence. This is an exercise to deepen and lose yourself in.

Guide Exercise 12:

Time: 30 min

Purpose: To activate Jing-energy in the body ❤ Activate the nerves ❤ Healing organs and glands

Preparation: Seated basic position, warm-up and a short inner smile.

1. Warm your hands by rubbing them against each other, put your hands over your breasts.

2. Connect with them by smiling at them and by feeling the breasts from the inside.

3. Put the tip of your tongue on the palate.

4. Direct your attention to the pineal gland while massaging around the nipples with your three middle fingers on each hand, outwards, slowly 10 turns (up the middle, out, down the sides). Feel the connection down to the clitoris and how it activates the pineal gland inside the head when you massage around your nipples. Pause for a while but keep your focus on the pineal gland.

5. Then return the attention to your breasts and your heart. Now massage inwards, 10 turns (down middle, out, up the sides)

6. Then, direct attention to the pituitary gland, as with the pineal gland. Feel the connection, focus behind and in between the eyebrows. Massage your nipples outwards and then pause.

7. Then massage inwards again and focus back on the breasts and heart.

8. Continue in this same way with all the glands: thyroid, thymus, pancreas, adrenals and ovaries.

9. Finish by laying your hands, palms up, on your knees. Focus on the breasts and the heart center and the energy you have collected there. Let the energy expand out into your body.

10. Then direct the energy down to the sexual center.

11. Make the SC or the last part of the hormone shower exercise (where you guide the energy up through the central channel, Chong Mai, and let the energy squirt out like a fountain).

12. Finish by collecting the energy in Dan Tian and have a soft focus on the heart center.

13. Rest for at least 10-15 minutes.

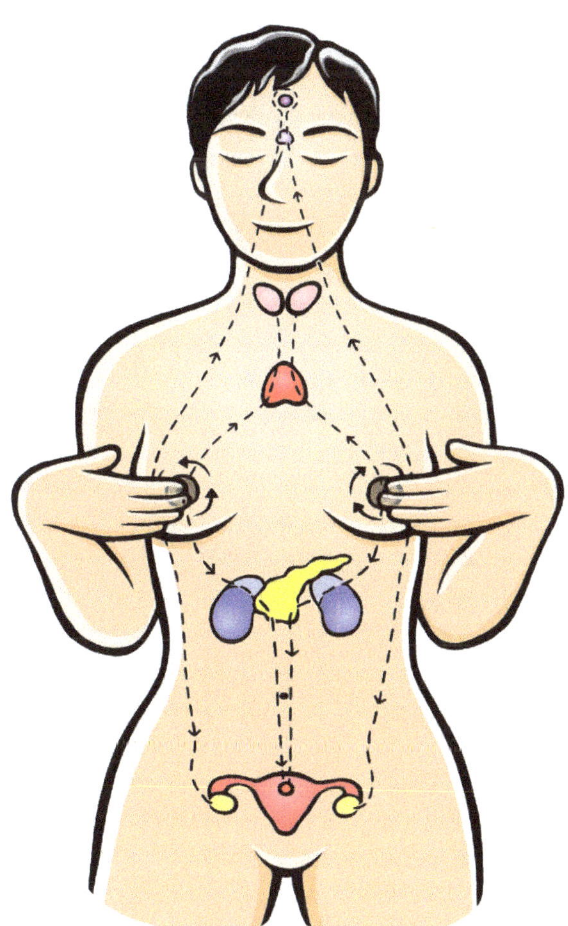

Massage the breasts around the nipples with the three middle fingers, while mentally directing the energy to the glands. Mixing sexual and hormone Jing Qi.

EXERCISE 13:

Squeezing exercises

The pelvic floor is made up of different, overlapping layers of muscles and fascia, which can be resembled to several hammocks suspended in different layers and in various directions. The muscles cooperate to keep everything in place and form a floor to support the genitals and the organs in the abdomen. They are assigned to regulate the opening and closing of the urethra, vagina and anus. They play an important roll in supporting women's sexual respons and affect the erogenous zones and contract during orgasm. As this floor awaken to its full capacity it hold the very foundation of both your spiritual and sexual potential.

Why train the pelvic floor muscles?

A strong and flexible pelvic floor is good to have for several reasons. The most important thing is to prevent incontinence, both urinary and anal, and to support internal organs. Healty muscles also favor vaginal lubrication and help the secretion during arousal to flow and facilitates orgasm and ejaculation. Unfit pelvic floor muscles can be the reason for different reproductive and sexual health problems. According to Tao, the pelvic floor muscles also balance the rest of the muscles throughout the body and strengthen your body's grounding and connection to the earth.

It's not only important to be able to tighten your pelvic floor muscles. Just as with other muscles in the body, it is equally important to be able to relax them. Relaxation is needed for the blood to reach and oxygenate all the cells. Both overly tense or too weak muscles decrease blood flow, as well as the flow of Qi along the meridians in the pelvic floor. Over time, this can create imbalances that can eventually lead to ill health. If the muscles are too tense it can also affect the orgasmic nerves. It can lead to less pleasure, numbness and even pain. Many women has problem with recurrent urinary tract infection (UTI). To tense pelvic floor can be the reason, because the lack of circulation creates a weakened urethral environment. Then the UTI is not caused by bacteria and the antibiotics will not work. Tense muscles can also be involved in bladder infection.

By exercising the muscles of the pelvic floor, your strength, agility and sensitivity can develop. Women often experience a deep sense of joy and love as the pelvic floor relaxes and the sex is awakened to its full potential. Recapturing the ability to orgasm gives a strong sense of satisfaction. Self-love and gratitude for one's own body usually come as a natural consequence.

Reasons for unfit pelvic floor

Often the pelvic floor and its muscles are a misunderstod or forgotten area, perhaps associated with pain or just embarrassing. Sometimes we miss that emotional stress may cause unconsciousness of the genital area. Most of us have at some time done or been exposed to something we did not wanted, that filled us with shame. Then we have a tendency to abandon ourselves and our body to protect ourselves from the unpleasant feeling. Stress and worry or feeling of not being enough make all the energy go up to the throat. It becomes difficult to ground, rest and find recovery in the body, to not mention the sex drive. The body tense up. We loose the contact with our pelvis and get unaware of the tension. A bad habit is created.

If you often had intercource which you did not want, or before you where ready, the muscles can react and want to protect you. If the reaction becomes automatic the tension may become cronic. It can result in pain during intercourse. It may be past trauma or abuse that left traces and symptoms. Also performance in bed, and attempts to create and push out an orgasm can trigger the muscles, as well as trying to hold back ejaculation.

Other causes may be poor posture or sedentary, childbirth, pregnance, menopause, injury, misery, loss of life, overwight etc. Cronic tension can cause "headache" in the pelvic floor. The good news is that whatever the cause of the tension is, the well-being will increase, by softening and exercise the pelvic floor.

Research

About one in three women cannot contract the muscles of the pelvic floor. And only 30% of all women can perform a proper contraction of the pelvic floor muscles after verbal instruction. Half have such a poor squeezing ability that the pressure in the urethra is not affected. There is evidence that weak pelvic floor muscles are a common factor, primarily in various urine leakages, but also in prolapse, anal incontinence, sexual ailments and pains. Research has found there to be a positive effect on the sex life from doing pelvic floor exercises. Some studies show that women who can ejaculate have shown that they rarely suffer from incontinence. According to recent studies, the pelvic floor muscles also work in synergy with the deep torso muscles. By chance, researchers have discovered that after a period of back pain with accompanying stabilization training, elite athletes no longer experience urine leakage. This mainly applies to stress urinary incontinence (SUI), which is when urine leaks out when there's sudden pressure on the bladder and urethra.

Core stability and abdominal pressure

Stabilizing the abdomen is about strengthening all the muscles surrounding the organs in the abdominal cavity. The pelvic floor muscles form the floor, the diaphragm is the ceiling, the walls around it consist of muscles in the abdomen and back. The muscle that has mainly been linked to incontinence is the transverse abdominal muscle, which sits like a girdle around the whole abdominal area. Together with the other muscles, it is constantly working to keep the chest up and is therefore very important for your posture. Abdominal pressure is created by simultaneous contractions of the abdominal and back muscles, the diaphragm and the pelvic floor. You can feel it when you, for example, cough, laugh, sneeze, sing, empty your bladder or lift something heavy. The easiest way to strengthen the transverse abdominal muscle is by simply breathing deeply. You can feel the muscle if you breathe down into your belly and then hiss the air out slowly. While doing so the lower part of the stomach should deflate. In conjunction with the egg exercises further ahead, you're not only training your pelvic floor but also your core stability.

Does it pay off to exercise?

There is convincing evidence that the pelvic floor exercise has a good effect on urinary incontinence. Hundreds of studies show that only three months of training shows results. Up to 70% of the participants in the surveys noted improvements while performing the exercises correctly. Muscle strength requires consistent practice and can quickly be

The pelvic floor seen from below

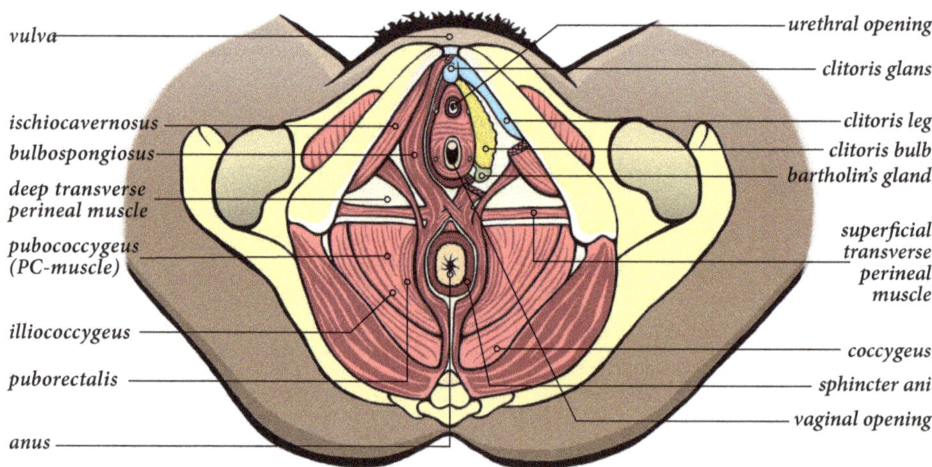

trained if you exercise regularly. Muscle strength is fresh produce. The recommendation is to also practice preventatively and not wait until issues arise. Common mistakes that women make are that they don't exercise often enough or that they practice in the wrong way. Few can manage to isolate the squeezes from the beginning, and require technical knowledge and awareness of which muscles are affected. But with the right guidance, most can learn both quickly and easily.

How should I exercise?

The first step is to get a better feel for how the pelvic floor functions and to find the muscles. Study the anatomy and try to feel the muscles in yourself. A complete training program should then include strength, speed and endurance training, as well as sensitivity training and relaxation. Since surveys have shown that it is difficult to learn effective squeezing techniques, guidance and some form of feedback is the best help. Vaginal weights, such as stone eggs, can sometimes be helpful.

Which muscles is it?

The pelvic floor consists of two layers of muscle, the pelvic diaphragm and urogenital diaphragm and at the bottom sphincters around the urethra, vagina and anus.

The pelvic diaphragm

These muscles run horizontally from the tailbone to the pubic bone and surrounds the urethra, vaginal and anal duct. The diaphragm forms two upward reaching arches and is situated at the top of the pelvis, that is, the deepest part of the vagina. They form a bowl. These hammock-like arches flatten out when the muscles are contracted and by doing so they close the openings. You can raise the entire pelvic floor, stop your urine and prevent incontinence. The muscle stimulates the vaginal walls and thereby also the prostate, G-zone and A-zone. The pelvic diaphragm is the largest muscle group with levator ani as its main muscle. Levator ani in turn, consists of three main parts, of which the most significant one is the pubococcygeus (PC muscle) that lies adjacent to the vagina. The other parts of the levator ani are the puborectalis, iliococcygeus and sometimes, even a fourth, the coccygeus, is counted to belong to these.

Urogenital diaphragm

The urogenital diaphragm is triangular shaped with the base at the sitting bones and the top point at the pubic bone, located inferior to the pelvic diaphragm and in the front part of the pelvis. It is sometimes called the perineal membrane and includes the deep and superficial transverse perineal muscles. The muscle permeates and stabilizes the root of the vaginal wall, and both the urethra and vagina penetrate it.

Sphincter muscles

Around the vagina and urethra is the bulbospongiosus muscle, which covers the clitoris bulbs and stimulates them during squeezing. Around the anus is the sphincter ani and around the urethra is the sphincter urethra. These are located at the bottom of the pelvic floor at the openings. Further to the sides is also the ischiocavernosus, which covers the clitoris legs.

Test your pelvic floor muscles

How do I know if I have an excessively weak or tight muscle?

Test: Can you stop the stream by squeezing when you pee?
If you can't stop the urine flow or if you find it difficult to, you probably have weak muscles, or an ignorance of how to best use them.

Finger test: Insert a finger into your vagina, about 2-3 inches. Use oil or lube if needed. Squeeze your finger with your muscles and judge by how it feels.

- Can't squeeze the finger = loose
  If the opening is very loose and open, and you can't squeeze the finger, or only a little, the muscle is weak.

- Can squeeze the finger = resilient
  A resilient, strong and healthy muscle can squeeze the finger noticeably and can also relax.

- Can't insert the finger = tense
  If you can't insert your finger, the muscle is very tense. Try massaging the tense muscles of the vaginal opening, and press them down towards the anus to soften them. You may then direct your breathing down towards your pelvic floor and ask for it to relax. Gradually massage the muscles from inside the vagina.

The squeezing exercises and numbers (turns, time) which follow are various suggestions of training. Perform fewer exercises or spend less time on them if you are having a hard time, and then increase as your strength increases. Regular training gives results. Take note of your strengths and weaknesses.

- It's better to make a few dozen squeezes a day than none at all.

- Try to only flex your pelvic floor muscles and relax your abdomen, buttocks, thighs etc.

- There are many occasions in everyday life for training such as standing in line, on the bus, in front of the tv etc. No one can see what you're doing.

Guide exercise 13:

Time: 10-15 min

Purpose: Find the muscles ❤ Practice strength and relaxation ❤ Raise awareness of flexibility and sensitivity

Preparation: Basic position, standing warm-up, especially ”open hip”, where you wiggle and circle the tailbone, to activate the pelvic floor. Then start by just squeezing to find and feel the muscle. Notice how it feels and what happens when you squeeze. Always relax after each squeeze.

1. Easy squeeze exercise

This simple squeeze exercise helps a weak muscle to become stronger and tense muscles to relax.

- Squeeze for 5 seconds and relax for 5 seconds. It's just as important to relax as to squeeze. Do this 10 squeezes, 3 times a day. Increase the number as it gets easier.

- Goal: 30 squeezes per session, three times a day, five days a week until you are strong.

2. Get to know your pelvic floor muscles

Strength and relaxation:

- Squeeze on inhalation and relax on exhalation. Do this 10 times.

- Squeeze exhalation and relax on inhalation. Do this 10 times.

- Squeeze and hold for 10 seconds regardless of breathing, relax for 10 seconds. Do this 3 times.

Endurance and speed:

- Squeeze 20 times, as fast as you can.

- Squeeze as hard as you can and hold on inhalation. Do this 3 times.

- Squeeze as hard as you can and hold on exhalation. Do this 3 times.

Sensitivity:

- Try to squeeze soft, hard, fast, slow. Feel what type of squeezing it is that activate the most sensation and energy for you. Don't think about breathing.

- Squeeze on inhalation with a sucking sensual feeling up through the vagina. Can you also sense and touch the vaginal walls and the cervix?

- Yoni breathing: To make this sensual squeezing above even more beautiful and juisy you can imagine that you are sucking up nurturing energy up through the vagina, like through a straw, on the inhalation. On the exhalation, you fill the entire womb space with pleasure and awaken your erotic genital body parts. Sit and build subtile sexual energy for several minutes.

Pelvic floor awareness:

- Squeeze the muscles around the clitoris and vagina. You can feel this right below the pubic bone.

- Squeeze the muscles around the anus. You can feel this at the tailbone.

- Squeeze the muscles at the perineum. You can feel this between the anus and the vagina.

- Squeeze the muscles on the left side and then the right side of the vaginal opening. You can feel this at the sitting bone. Activate the muscles by pressing the respective footpad against floor if you lie down or sit. If you stand, push down with your toes.

- Squeeze only the muscles in the lower part of the pelvic floor (around the vagina and anal opening). Then the middle urogenital triangle in the front, and then the pelvic diaphragm, that goes from tail to pubic bone in the highest part of the pelvic floor. You can squeeze them all like an elevator going up 3 levels, and then going down, and relax.

Sexual genital fitness

Genital fitness is promoting sexual health, self-confidence and enhancing sexual fulfillment. To get there you need to take charge over your pelvic floor muscles. You can even learn to stimulate a penis, while the man is remaining passive, only by using the pelvic floor muscles. This is an ancient love art and technique from Asia, in Hindu tradition called pompoir. This means being able to use the different muscles, know the different levels, from the vagina opening and up the canal to cervix, and different kinds of squeezings, like; sucking, sucking in waves, pulsing, rapid squeezes, slow puls, push out, pull in, hold firm etc. You can add these different ways and qualities of squeezing to the pelvic floor exercises.

With a good practice you tone the vaginal walls when the blood flow and Qi increase. Nerves can work better when the muscles get more resilient, which lead to hightened presence, sensitivity and pleasure. And as if that wasn't enough, you become a greater and more sucessfull lover.

Stone egg exercises

The custom to strengthen the vagina, using a stone egg, comes from ancient China. From the beginning, it was only taught in the royal palace to promote good health, youth and a resilient and moist vagina. The exercises strengthen the pelvic floor muscles, the Qi-muscle or orgasm-muscle, as the Taoist call it. In this manner you improve your capacity to lift energy up along the spine and to distribute it among the organs, glands and brain. This exercise can create deep healing and improve your ability to guide energy. This is also a beneficial restorative practice after childbirth.

Weak pelvic floor muscles result in leakage of life energy, as well as weak pelvic organs, which then hang down and press against the perineum. If the muscle is resilient, the pelvic floor can work as a good support for the organs and can prevent life energy from escaping unnecessarily.

The strength of the muscle requires constant upkeep. If you don't use it, you will lose it. Muscles quickly lose their strength without practice, but are luckily quick to train. Do the muscle test before you start on p. 130. What's most effective is to choose a specific program and perform it regularly.

The advantage of practicing with an egg is that you'll feel more and can give better feedback to yourself. A smaller egg is harder to hold in place than a larger one. Start with a larger egg if you think you have a weak pelvic floor muscle. And of course adapt the size depending on how tight or wide you are. Preferably use a stone egg made of jade, or another natural stone, with a drilled hole through it. This makes it possible for you to attach a string to the egg and hold on to it when you squeeze. Use dental floss, which is both strong and hygienic, or side thread. Some will also attach weights to the string as the muscle strength increases. These exercises using an egg are sometimes called "ovarian Kung Fu".

- All of the following exercises can be performed with or without an egg.

- You can also perform the aforementioned squeezing exercises with an egg.

- Be careful when inserting the egg into the vagina. Check to feel that you're ready and use lubricant if you need to. Warm the egg in your hands before inserting it.

- It may be difficult to feel the egg in the beginning. Use your finger to feel how high up it is. Insert it and push it up using your finger, then relax for it to slide down. Then squeeze and tighten the muscle and try to notice when the egg goes up. Check and look how the string move up and down.

- You can have the egg inserted when you're at home for a few hours. This will stimulate the flow in the vaginal walls. Sense the egg and keep part of your awareness in the vagina.

- If you are unable to hold the egg in place, start with doing the exercises in a lying position or practice without an egg.

- To prevent from only building yang and strength, remember to relax after each contraction to also nurture your yin-nature and receptivity.

- Do some warm-up exercises, especially hip-movement where you wiggle and circle the tailbone, to activate the pelvic floor, before practise egg exercises.

Note

- Do not perform the egg exercises if you are on your period, are pregnant or have an acute infection or an intrauterine system (IUS). If you for some reason want to try this anyway, be careful and gentle.

- If you suspect that you have very tense muscles, do not use an egg. Be careful with the squeezing and focus first on relaxation. The muscle may just be cramping up and squeezing can make it worse.

Egg care

Boil the egg for five minutes before using it for the first time, to guarantee that it's clean and free of bacteria. Put the egg in when the water is cold. After boiling it the first time it's enough to just wash the egg with soap between uses. You can always boil the egg again if needed.

Lying egg exercise

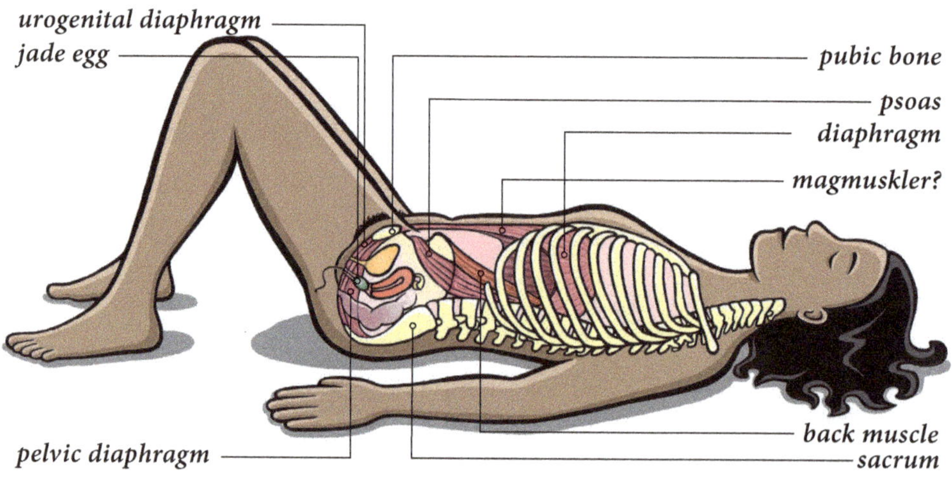

Guide exercise 14:

Time: 10 min, standing or lying down

Purpose: To increase the production of secretions, to obtain smooth mucous membranes and to counteract bacteria ❤ Develop both strength and sensitivity in the pelvic floor ❤ Open up your vagina, your inner heart

Preparation: Standing or lying basic position and warm-up, especially "open hip", where you wiggle and circle the tailbone, to activate the pelvic floor, and a short inner smile.

Lying egg exercises

Attach a string to the egg and gently insert it into your vagina. How much can you resist when pulling on the string? Notice how strong you are.

1. Lie on your back with bent knees and with the soles of your feet on the floor. Angle your tailbone and sacrum upwards on inhalation and squeeze the egg. The lumbar spine stays on the floor. Return your tail and sacrum down to the starting position on the exhale and relax. Use this moment to release all the tensions and, during the relaxation, guide them down to Mother Earth. Start calmly and gently. Then rock your tail and sacrum rhythmically up and down for a few minutes. Stretch your legs out and rest. Then try the same movement as above, but with reverse breathing. Roll up on the exhalation and roll it down on the inhalation and relax.

2. Lie on your back with bent knees and the soles of your feet on the floor. Inhale and slowly roll up the spine, one vertebra at the time. Hips go up toward the ceiling. At the same time, do a sucking squeeze up through the vagina, from the opening to the cervix. Roll up as far as you can and press your hips toward the ceiling. Exhale and slowly roll down vertebra after vertebra. Hips come down to the floor again. Relax and release the squeeze on the way down. Do this 3 times.

3. Lie on your back, bend your legs and lift your knees to your chest and hold your knees there with your arms. Exhale, squeeze, lift the tailbone, then the sacrum, push the lumbar spine down against the floor, come up with your upper chest slightly and hold. Inhale and come down. Do this 5 times.
    Then let your knees fall to the sides so that it stretches your groin and opens your genital region, then put the soles of the feet together and rest.

4. Then do the same movement as before, no. 3, but faster. On exhalation, when you come up, you simultaneously squeeze the vagina and anus along with your eyes and your mouth, as hard as you can. The sphincter muscles in the face and genitals are connected. Get down quickly and then up again. Squeeze 10 times. Stretch out flat and rest.

Standing egg exercises

Attach a string to the egg and gently insert it into your vagina. Can you feel the egg? How much awareness do you have in your vagina? How much can you resist when pulling the string? Notice how strong you are.

1. Stand in a standing basic position. Squeeze the egg and inhale, and simultaneously move the tailbone forward, in between the legs, tilt the pelvis backwards and the arch of the lower back disappears. Come back on the exhale: the tailbone comes back and you can arch your back slightly again and relax. Do this 10 times.

Do the same with reverse breathing. Exhale and squeeze when the tailbone is tucked in between the legs and the pelvis is tilted backwards. Inhale and relax as you go back. Notice the difference.

Do standing egg exercise with firebreath

When you do fire breathing, you breathe vigorously, in and out of the nose. On exhalation, the belly is emptied of air and the navel quickly moves backwards and inwards towards Ming Men, in the lumbar spine. On the inhale the belly and navel move forward. Practice only the fire breathing first. The fire gives the internal organs a beneficial massage. The point is to also learn how to control the big breathing muscle, the diaphragm. Before you get used to it, perform the fire breathing soft and gently.

2. Then do the fire breathing with a squeeze and the pelvic movements above, no. 1. Inhale and squeeze when the tailbone is tucked in. In the beginning, perform the hip movement, soft and gently and then more and more powerful.
    Then do the same with reverse fire breathing. Exhale and squeeze when the tailbone is tucked in. This last movement will help prevent stress urinary incontinence.

- Once you have done these exercises a number of times, try to estimate if your strength has increased by squeezing the egg and holding it while pulling the string. Also note if your sensitivity and awareness have increased?

- If it feels too cumbersome to squeeze on different breaths, do the type of breathing that feels most natural in the beginning.

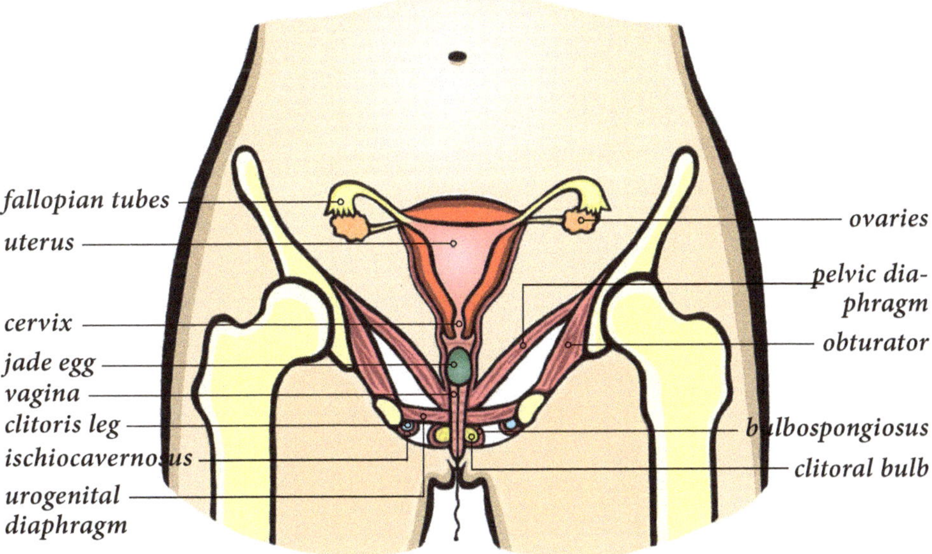

Finish with removing the egg by:

- Just relax and let the egg slip out. If necessary, help pushing the egg out using your muscles or pull it out using the string.

- Squatting and pushing or coughing.

- Lie on your back on the floor, lift your legs up, and let your toes end up on the floor behind your head. The butt should now be pointing straight up. In this position, push the egg out using your pelvic floor muscles and allow it to roll down the chute, formed by the back of your legs. This helps invigorate the ejaculation motion of the pelvic floor muscles, and it is fun.

Sit down, or lie down, and relax after the egg exercises, yin-phase. Receive the impact and feel all the Qi that has been built up. Be aware of your vagina, uterus and heart center. Enjoy the stillness in meditation or use the energy generated in some pleasurable way.

Stone egg ceremonies

A ceremony is a ritual, an act, with a symbolic meaning. It has a clear intention to guide the energy in a certain direction.

Caring for the womb

The womb is a powerful energy source with an ability that goes far beyond giving birth. The uterus is very sensitive and receptive. It not only absorbs your personal knowledge and experiences but also the collective impressions. This often happens unconsciously though. Years of negative emotions may have accumulated and poisoned your uterus. Unconsciousness or unwillingness to feel certain emotions has ultimately led to breaking this power and your connection to your womb, and thus the connection to your instincts and feminine essence. It is time for all women to heal and regain the power of the full womb space. These exercises and ceremonies below support and empower this recapturing.

Your creational power

The Jing energy is strongly associated with your life force energy, creativity and creative ability. The ovaries symbolically keep the seeds of all possibilities and it is in your uterus that everything takes shape, including your life projects and your dreams. Like a womb space with a fertile soil which you can nourish and make seeds grow and take form. Take good care of these seeds and take the time to find out what really hides behind your needs and what you truly long for. Find your own motivation and notice what is really important to you. Then let your dreams be fertilized by your thirst for life and ability to direct your energy. In sexual magic, you take your intentions and allow them to mate with the most powerful energy we have, the sexual orgasmic energy. How do you perceive this potent energy and how do you want to use your orgasmic creational power? How do you create space for the new to take shape?

Egg exercise as a purification ceremony

Ask the egg to help with cleansing yourself and your genitals from thoughts, feelings, memories and experiences that no longer serve you. Then insert the egg. Call upon and inhale the experiences and emotions you want out of your system. When you exhale you fill the egg with these emotions and memories. The egg must be made out of a natural mineral to be able to store the energy inside. Then pull the egg out and everything you filled it with. Feel and imagine how all the energies you no longer need leave you when you extract the egg. Then fill yourself with the new, all that which you want to allow into your life.

Do not forget to clean the egg properly after this exercise. For example, in the sun, in the moonlight, in a glass of salt water or bury the egg in the earth for a while.

An egg ceremony for your dream

Ask the egg to hold a dream that you have, an intention, something you want to create in your life, birth and bring into life. Insert the egg and imagine that you are sowing a seed into your fertile womb space. Perform any of the egg exercises as usual. Let your desire take shape in your interior, in the yin phase. Take out and thank the egg and ask your dream to come true and be manifested. Please do this little ceremony on several occasions for the same life project.

Creative expression

These small ceremonies can be combined to great advantage with creative expressions. It can be writing down your experiences or desires, painting them, making a collage or an altar with the new things you want to create in the future. The manifestation process is about turning a future dream into reality in the present. A sense of that your wish has already been realized. You can also strengthen your dreams by sending your wish into the universe with your orgasm, the creative power itself.

Training tips

It's better to practice 15 minutes per day than one hour, one day a week. Your Qi grows through regularity and you break patterns by acquiring new habits. These are techniques that you practice over time rather than temporary experiences. Pick out a couple of exercises at a time to immerse yourself in. Gain experience by at least training three times a week for three months. Then you get an idea and feel for what an exercise can give you and if it works. Regular practice will for sure speed up your evolution. A clear intention gives you extra power in the exercise and raises your motivation. Don't forget that the yin phase is an important part of the practise.

Example of practice sequence

The basic training is the inner smile and the small circulation. Begin by balancing your emotions, cultivating self-acceptance and learning how to circulate energy. If you need to ground yourself then do the exercise with The Tree. If you want to balance or explore your hormone system, you perform breast massage, charge your life energy, perform a hormone shower or gland exercise. If you have a weak pelvic floor or would like to elevate your orgasticness, you focus on the squeezing and egg exercises. In ovary breathing, you exercise your life energy, as well as lifting vital energy up through your spine.

Preparation is always the basic position, exercise 1, and preferably the warm-up exercises, exercise 2, and/or a short inner smile, exercise 6. Finishing up is done by collecting the energy, exercise 3.

Suggestions for exercise combinations

The tree and the inner smile (exercise 4 + 5).

The inner smile and the small circulation (exercise 5 + 7).

Charge your life energy, ovary breathing and the small circulation (exercise 9 + 10 + 7).

Short inner smile and hormone shower (exercise 6 + 11).

Gland exercise and small circulation (exercise 12 + 7).

Breast massage and egg exercise (exercise 8 + 14).

Magic tools

You can view all exercises as magic tools for growth or as a means of transportation to help you even further in your path through life. In the beginning, you guide your energy, but you will eventually learn to just follow your natural current. Mastering a technique is not what's important here, but empowering yourself and finding just as much space for self-reflection and rest in everyday life as you need. A place to which you can return and gather life energy and create health and well-being. Keep in mind that you are unique and valuable and can choose to say yes to cultivating your feminine beauty and radiance.

*Good luck with your practice and
the development of your full potential!*

HORMONE WORDLIST

Here is a brief presentation of some of the most important hormones and their properties in this context. Different substances trigger different functions, expressions and behavor. Estrogen, for example, is called the queen because of her feminine qualities.

Adrenaline

A stress hormone stimulated by the sympathetic nervous system. Kicks off in danger, physical exertion, mental stress and anger. Coffee stimulates adrenaline. Is a neurotransmitter excreted from the adrenal glands.

Aldosterone

An adrenal hormone that regulates blood pressure and fluid balance. May be involved in the creation of female ejaculation. Stimulated by the sympathetic nervous system.

Androgens

Male sex hormones, the most common are testosterone and DHEA.

Cortisol

A steroid and a stress hormone that play an important role, though indirectly, in sexual response. High level diminishes interest in sex. Released to counter stress, fear and inflamation. High levels of long-term stress can have devastating consequences on both the immune system and the psyche. Balance and the right level are important for metabolism. Excreted from the adrenals.

DHEA (dehydroepiandrosterone)

Is the mother of most sex hormones and pheromones and is the hormone we have the most of in the body. A well-being and rejuvenating hormone that has several positive effects. It does not decrease during menopause and is considered important because it can convert to sex hormones. It is involved in your sexuality and orgasm. Produced in the adrenals, but also in the brain and gonads. Qigong, meditation and moderate sunbathing increases DHEA.

DMT (dimethyltryptamine)

Similar to serotonin and is found naturally in the pineal gland. Exact function is unknown, but is one of the psychedelic ingredients in ayahuasca. It is found in several teacher plants and is used in South America for healing and growing. Probably important for our dreaming and our creativity.

Dopamine

Without this hormone we would not feel joy or enthusiasm. It is a rewarding hormone, linked to love, euphoria and desire. Involved in many addictions, from alcohol to cocaine. It is also what makes us go for anything we desire. Deficiency can cause depression and heaviness. Is excreted from the pineal gland, stimulate oxytocine and is a precursor to noradrenaline.

Endorphins

The body's natural pain relievers and depression lifters. The hormone affects our desire to sleep, eat and drink. Endorphin is secreted by laughter, stress, exercise, but also by sex and love. A rewarding hormone linked to physical well-being and euphoria. Secreted from the hypothalamus.

Estrogene

The most female hormone of them all. Makes you soft, sensitive, receptive, attractive and willing. Is a group of female hormones; estriol, estradiol and estrone. Regular sexual activity increases the presence and change your overall hormone chemistry and therefore how you look at life. Forms in the ovaries, adrenals, brain and fat cells on command from the pituitary gland.

Glucagon

Excreted at lower blood sugar levels. Opposite to insulin. Increases mobilization of stored energy supplies. Increases also by hard work or starvation. Excreted by the pancreas.

Insulin

Excreted after meal when blood sugar is raised. Impaired function or insensitivity to the hormone is called diabetes. Glucagon, adrenaline and noradrenaline counteract the insulin. Formed in the pancreas.

Melatonin

The amount varies during the day and is affected by the light. Levels increase during the night. Some believe that it increases our libido, affects depression and improves sleep. Has antioxidant effect and strengthens the immune system. Is produced by the pineal gland via the serotonin.

Neurotransmitters

Messenger that is mediated through nerve signals and secreted into the blood via nerve pathways. Can be dopamine, adrenaline and serotnin.

Noradrenaline

A stress hormone that is important for the sympathetic nervous system. Raises the bood pressure och increases the cardiac activity. Intensifies alertness, enthusiasm and concentration. Deficiency can create hopelessness. Is both a neurotransmitter and a blood-borne hormone. Secreted from adrenals and pineal gland.

Oxytocin

Increases through touch and is important for us to want to be united with a partner. Just the thought of a lover can raise the levels. It initiates contractions in the pelvic floor during both orgasm and delivery and maximum levels occur just after. The hormone decreases stress and increases wellbeing. A neurohormone that is triggered from pituitary gland and hypthalamus.

PEA (phenethylamine)

A love hormone that makes you euphoric or romantic. It is naturally in your flow when you are in love. At most during orgasm and makes you love sick if it dips. It reduces your hunger. Speeds up the flow of information between cells and gives hightened awareness. A neurotransmitter found in the brain. Avaliable in chocolate.

Pheromones

Substances that we secrete to affect others through our scent. It's scents are very important for our choice of partners. Originated from DHEA.

Progesterone

Female sex hormone who are not so versed in sex and decreases the pheromones. They increase their presence the weeks after ovulation and decreases radically shortly before the period starts. If you get pregnant it makes you calm, caring and protective. The balance with the estrogen seem to be important. Imbalance can affect mood and cause PMS. It is produced mainly in the ovaries and adrenals.

Prolactin

Increases during pregnancy and breastfeeding and then the sex drive decreases. Can increase by orgasm, but decreases fast. Linked to the immune system, mental health and metabolism. Also increses by stimulating the cervix, physical workout and stress. Secrets from the pituitary.

Relaxin

Causes the cervix and the pelvic floor to relax. Also affects the secretion of aldosterone. Comes from the ovaries.

Serotonin

A hormone with two faces. Can make you shy or more assertive, depending on level. Some mean that the right level makes you fall in love. High levels cool down your libido, but makes you sensitive and peaceful. Low level intensifies desire, accelerates orgasm, and you can even become agressive. Triggers the oxytocin. Secreted from the pineal gland.

Sex hormones

Estrogens, progesterone, testosterone.

Steroid hormones

Created from cholesterol. Could be DHEA, testosterone, estrogene, progesteron or cortisol.

Stress hormones

Adrenaline, noradrenaline and cortisol.

Testosterone

Male and pleasurable characteristics with a dominant undertone. Makes you take the initiative and wanting to have sex, mark the territory and protect. Help building the muscles and strengthen the skeleton. Formed in the ovaries and adrenals.

Thyroid hormones

Thoraxin, but is termed T3 and T4. Increases metabolism and energy consumption. God for digestion, fertility and fat loss.

REFERENCES

Books about Tao and Tantra

Chang, Stephen T. (1992): The Tao of sexology: The Book of infinite wisdom. Tao publ.

Chia, Mantak et al. (2005): The Multi-orgasmic couple: Sexual secrets every couple should know. San Francisco: HarperOne.

Chia, Mantak et al. (2005): The Multi-orgasmic woman: How any woman can experience ultimate pleasure and dramatically enhance her health and happiness. USA: Rodale.

Désilets, Saida (2006): Emergence of the sensual woman: Awakening our erotic innocence: The sacred teaching of the jade goddess. Kihei: Goddess Publishing.

Lai, Hsi (2001): The sexual teachings of the white tigress: Secrets of the female Taoist masters. Vermont: Destiny Books.

Pawson, P. (1978): The art of Tantra. New York: Thames and Hudson.

Piontek, M. (2001): Exploring the hidden power of female sexuality: A workbook for women. York Beach: Weiser Books.

Richardson, Diana (2004): Tantric orgasm for women. Vermont: Inner Traditions.

Books about sexuality

Geels A. & Roos L. (red.).(2010). Sex – för guds skull: Sexualitet och erotik i världens religioner. [Sex - for God's sake: Sexuality and eroticism in the world's religions]. Lund: Studentlitteratur.

Charles, Amara (2011): The sexual practices of Quodoushka. Rochester: Destiny Books.

Franzén, Ylva (2007): Orgasmera mera: Vägar till kvinnlig njutning [Orgasm more: ways to female pleasure]. Stockholm: Xstory.

Hulter, Birgitta (2004): Sexualitet och hälsa. [Sex and health]. Lund: Studentlitteratur.

Komisaruk, Barry R. et al. (2002): The Science of orgasm. Baltimore: The John Hopkins University Press.

Nilsson, M & Wulcan, S. (2019): Kvinnlig ejakulation: Ett omdebatterat fenomen: En genealogisk diskursanalys. [Female ejaculation: A debated phenomenon]. Malmö: University.

Sexologi: [Sexology]: (2010, 3:e uppl.): Under red. av P.O. Lundberg. Stockholm: Liber.

Sundahl, Deborah (2014): Female ejaculation and the G-spot: Not your mother's orgasm book. New York: Turner Publishing.

Tunneshende, M. (2001): Don Juan and the art of sexual energy: The rainbow serpent of the Toltecs. Vermont: Bear & Company.

Books about Qigong

Chia, Mantak et al. (1993): Awakening the healing light of the Tao. New York: Healing Tao Books.

Cleary, T. (red.). (1996): Immortal sisters: Secret teachings of Taoist women. Berkeley: North Atlantic Books.

Cohen, Kenneth S. (1999): The way of Qigong: The art and science of Chinese energy healing. New York: Ballantine Books.

Liu, S., Blank, J. (2011): Secrets of dragon gate: Ancient Taoist practices for health, wealth and the art of sexual yoga. New York: Penguin.

Mitchell, Damo (2002): Daoist nei gong: The philosophical art of change. London: Singing dragon.

Skarpste-Malmqvist, Ruta (2007): Dokument Qigong: Kraftfull väg till självläkning och ökad livskvalité: Bakgrund, effekter och forskningsresultat. [Document Qigong: Powerful approach to self-health and increased life quality: Background, effects and research results]. Fritsla, Förlagstryckeriet Vinterleken.

Yang, J. (2006): Qigong meditations: small circulation. Boston: YMAA.

Other Books

Bodanis, D. (2008): E= mc2: A biography of the world's most famous equation. London: Pan MacMillan.

Childre, Doc et al. (1999): The Hearthmath solution. San Francisco: Harper.

Crenshawm T. (1996): The alchemy of love and lust: How our sex hormones influence our relationships. New York: Pocket Books.

Frank, Lone (2009): Mindfield: How brain science is changing our world. London: Oneworld Publ.

Haug, E et al.(1993): Människans fysiologi. [Human physiology]. Stockholm: Liber utbildning: Universitetsförlaget.

Heden, M. Et al. (2007): Vill man så kan man: En litteraturstudie av viljans inverkan på kroppens läkande förmåga [If you want you can: A litterature study of the will affecting the healing ability of the body]. Malmö Högskola.

Lipton, B.H. (2005): The Biology of belief. Spånga, Sorena.

Mares, Théun (1999): The Toltec teachings: Volume III. 3rd ed. Athens: Renascent Legacy Press.

Sellman, S. (2000): Hormone heresy: What woman must know about their hormones. Tulsa: Get Well International.

Articles

Akuthota V., Nadler S.F. (2004). Core strengthening. Arch Phys Med Rehabil, 2004;Vol. 85 (3 Suppl 1):S 86–92.

Baskin L.S. m. . (1999). Anatomical studies of the human clitoris. The Journal of Urology, 1999 Sep;162(3 Pt2):1015-20.

Cartwrignt, R. m. . (2007). Do women with female ejaculation have detrusor over-activity? Journal of Sexual Medicine, 2007;4:1655-1658.

Casillas, A.R. (2009). The female prostate: The End of the controvesy. Newsulletin, s. 24-25, December 2009.

Gravina, G.L. m. . (2008). Measurement of the thickness of the urethrovaginal space in women with or without vaginal orgasm. Journal of Sexual Medicine, 2008;5: 610-618.

Gruenwald, I. (2007). Physiological changes in female genital sensation during sexual stimulation. Journal of Sexual Medicine, 2007;4:390-394.

Koole, J. (2003). Menopause – Curse or blessing. Deertraks, December. Lederman, E. (2010).

Lederman, E. (2010). The Myth of core stability. CPDO Ltd, London. Journal of Bodywork & Movement Therapies, 14, 84-98.

O'connell, H. (2005). Anatomy of the clitoris. The Journal of Urology. October, Vol. 174 (4 Pt 1): 1189-95.

O'connell, H. (2005). Clitoral anatomy in nulliparous, healthy, premenstrual volunteers using unenhanced magnetic resonance imaging. The Journal of Urology, 2005;June, Vol. 173, Issue 6, Pages 2060-2063.

Wimpissinger, F. M. . (2007). The female prostate revisited: Perineal ultrasound and bio- cemical studies of female ejaculate. Journal of Sexual Medicine, 2007;4:1388-1393.

Zaviacic, M. (2001). The female prostate: history, functional morphology and sexology Implications. Sexologies Archives.

Web references:

Brown, J.B. (2000). Studies on human reproduction. Ovarian activity and fertility and the Billings ovulation method. Melbourne. From: www.billingsmethod.com

Chua Chee A. (2002). Talk about the A-spot (pdf). 7th Asian Conference of Sexology. Singapore. From: www.aspot-pioneer.com

Frank, P. (1996). Här har du din nya kärlekszon.[Here is your new love-zon]. From: www.home.swipnet.se/~w-59099/ samlevn/Apunkt.htm

Jannini, E.A. et al. (2011): The new insights from one case of female ejaculation www.jsm.jsexmed.org/article/S1743-6095(15)33346-4/fulltext

Jannini, E.A et al (2014): Beoynd the G-spot: clitourethrovaginal complex anatomy in female orgasm. www.ncbi.nlm.nih.gov/pubmed/25112854

Lam, M. (2011) Womens health, estrogen dominance. From: www.drlam.com Lee, J. (2011). Natural hormone balance. From: www.johnleemd.com

Pastor, Z (2013). Female ejaculation orgasm vs. coital incontinence: a systematic review. h p://www.ncbi.nlm.nih.gov/pubmed/?term=female+ejaculation+vs+coital+incontine nce.

Salama, S. m. . (2014). Nature and origin of "squirting" in female sexuality. www.researchgate.net/publication/270052805_Nature_and_Origin_of_Squirting_in_Female_Sexuality

SBU:s styrelse och råd. (2000). Behandling av urininkontinens: Sammanfattning och slutsatser. Stockholm, Statens beredning för medicinsk utvärdering. Från: www.sbu.se

Sveriges Radio. (2014). sverigesradio.se/sida/artikel.aspx?programid=406& artikel=5989656 (about Jannini and the CUV-complex).

INDEX

LIST OF ILLUSTRATIONS

THANK YOU!

Thank's to my teachers and inspirers

I would like to honor and thank some of the most significant teachers for me, who have contributed in various ways by sharing their knowledge and wisdom.

❤ **Andrew Kenneth Fretwell** ❤ **www.wuji-gong.org**

Andrew who travels worldwide teaching Wuji Gong is inspiring humanity to awaken self-love by grounding and crystalizing the essence of self (SOUL) and integrating it within the body/mind.

Andrew is a great bodyworker and the founder of The OFT – Original Feeling Touch – an innovative healing modality. He also teaches Taoist alchemy as well as Taoist sexual practice. Universal Tao senior instructor.

❤ **David Verdesi** ❤ **www.davidverdesi.com**

David has devoted his life to the human potential, primarily through his exploration of Taoism, Tantra and shamanism. He has a rich and profound knowledge of Qigong and Taoism and its theory, science and training. A true source of inspiration of self-knowledge and pointing out the nature of the human potential.

❤ **Mantak Chia** ❤ **www.universal-tao.com**

Master Chia is a knowledgeable and practical teacher who has summarized the Taoist wisdom from various teachers and shared it through many books and taught it all over the world. He is the one who has brought several of the Taoists sexual Qigong practices to the West and calls his system of methods Universal Tao.

❤ Deborah Sundahl ❤ www.deborahsundahl.com

Deborah is a pioneer with over 35 years of groundbreaking contributions to the field of the female prostate, G-spot and female ejacuation. She is a passionate spokesperson for female sexuality.

She lectures and give workshops in North America and in Europe and teaching how to understand and integrate this erotic body – the prostate - in both men and women.

❤ Åsa Kullberg ❤ www.asakullberg.com

Åsa teaches with great passion and amazing clarity shamanic sexual wisdom, which is a ceremonial process to reconnect and remember the naturalness of who you are as a sexual human being. The teachings are based in a shamanic tradition, Quodoushka, from the Sweet Medicine Sundance Path. It also includes Shamanic Body Dearmoring, a two-week process that frees and expands the overall life force energy and stimulates vital health and happiness.

Thank's to others

I would like to thank Lisa Larsson for her tireless work, resulting in all the amazing illustrations. Johan Badh for doing the basic translation and then Deborah Sundahl for invaluable feedback on the text as well as Sara Broman. For excellent proofreading I would like to thank Kicki Pallin and Lucas Serby and then Ann-Sofie Hammarström Östergren for exemplary and professional work with the layout and cover. Special thanks to Andrew Fretwell for inspiration and quotes, Björn Westin for specialist review and Ann-Margret Kälfors for help with the Swedish text. Others I want to mention with thankfulness is Leja Jansson, Monika Swärd, Lotta Sjöberg and Kaisa Hansen, as well as all of you who have given feedback or supported this project. Thank you all!

Further information

Here you will find more information:

❤ Web: www.pelvicfloorawareness.com & www.bodycoach.nu

❤ Mail: info@bodycoach.nu

Other books published in English by Iréne Andersson:

❤ Create Health with Your Sexual Energy: A Tao Approach to Men's Well-Being

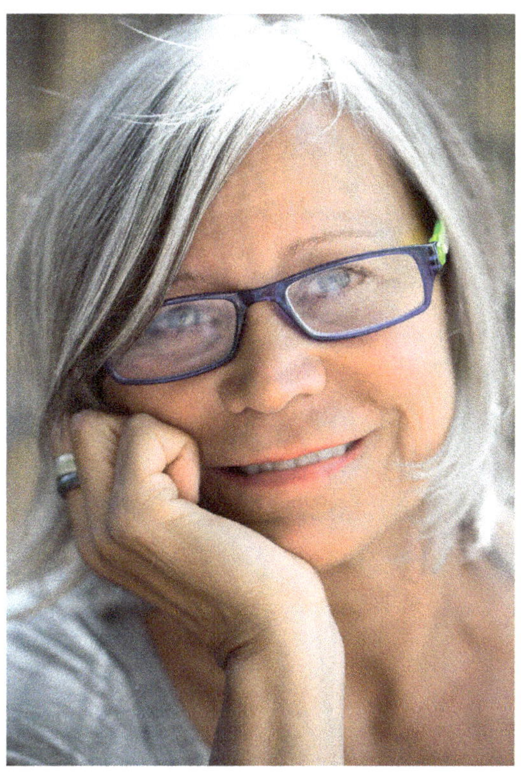

About Iréne Andersson

Iréne Andersson is from Sweden and has over 25 years of exploration and learning in different traditions and alternative methods, resulting in a unique combination of knowledge, experience and tools. Her specialty is Taoist sexual practice with focus on the pelvic floor and sexual health. She combines modern research with wisdom from different traditions of thought that has a holistic view. Iréne is a certified Qigong instructor since 1998 and has spent a lot of time with Taoist teachers in different countries, and also studied Tantra, Yoga and shamanism as well as psychological methods and school medicine. In a clinical setting, she offers pelvic floor treatment and bodywork, and gives trainings, workshops and lectures in pelvic floor awareness, sexual health and Taoist sexual practice.

www.pelvicfloorawareness.com

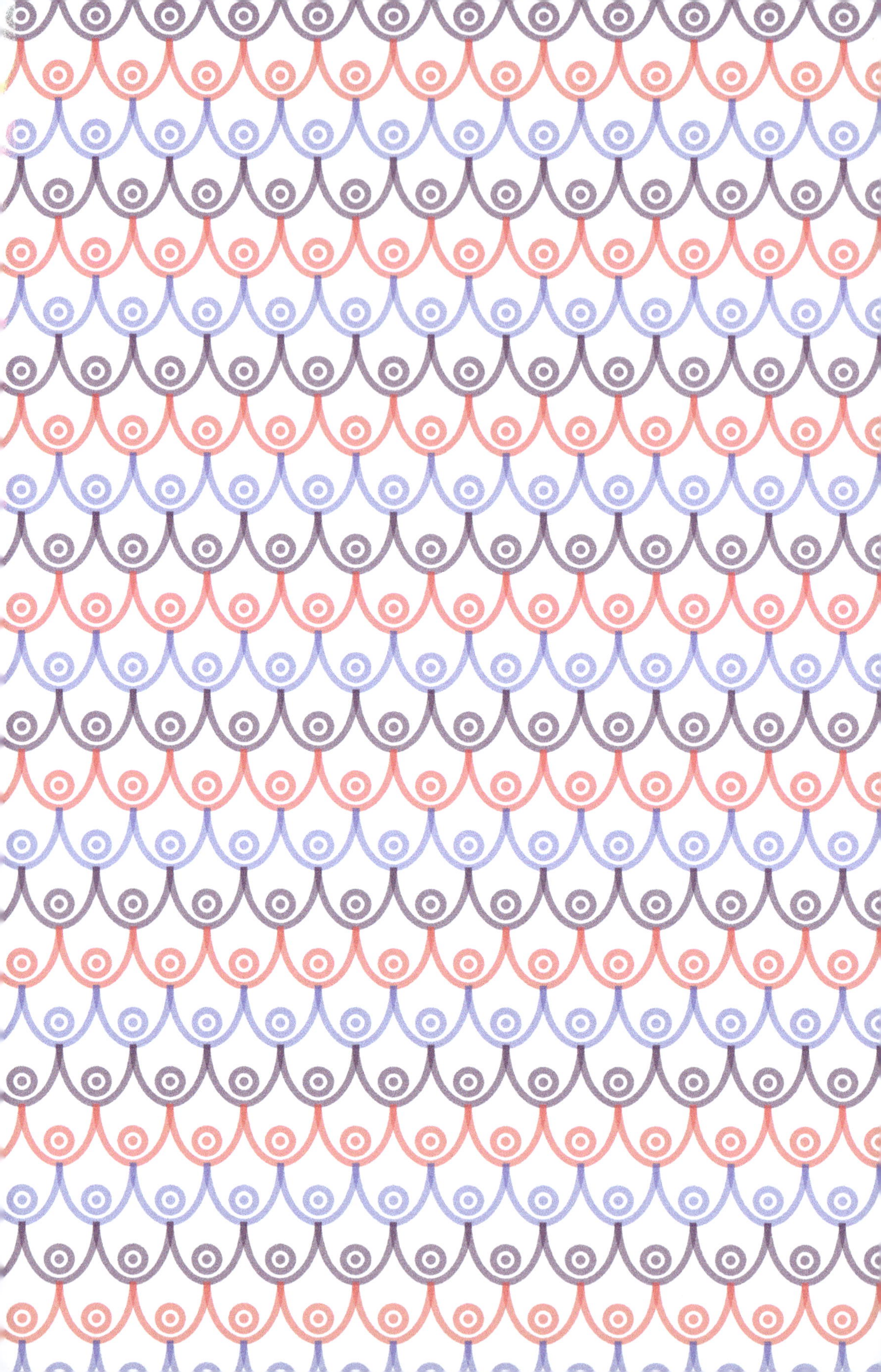